4/92

D0717268

COLOUR ATLAS
OF
MINOR SURGERY
IN
GENERAL PRACTICE

Presented to

----

with the compliments of

----

your Upjohn Representative

As a service to medical education | Upjohn |

COLOUR ATLAS OF MINOR SURGERY IN GENERAL PRACTICE

by

John Fry

General Practitioner

Ian Higton

General Surgeon

John Stephenson

Consultant ENT Surgeon

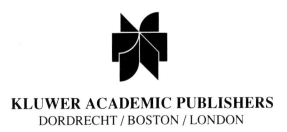

KLUWER ACADEMIC PUBLISHERS

DORDRECHT / BOSTON / LONDON

Distributors

for the United States and Canada : Kluwer Academic Publishers, P.O. Box 358, Accord Station, Hingham, MA 02018-0358, U.S.A.
for all other countries : Kluwer Academic Publishers Group, Distribution Center, P.O. Box 322, 3300 AH Dordrecht, The Netherlands

ISBN 0-7923-8945-X

Copyright

© 1990 by Kluwer Academic Publishers

All rights reserved. No part of this publication may be reproduced, stored in a retrieval system, or transmitted in any form or by any means, electronic, mechanical, photocopying, recording or otherwise, without prior permission from the publishers, Kluwer Academic Publishers BV, P.O. Box 17, 3300 AA Dordrecht, The Netherlands.

Published in the United Kingdom by Kluwer Academic Publishers, P.O. Box 55, Lancaster, U.K.

Kluwer Academic Publishers BV incorporates the publishing programmes of D. Reidel, Martinus Nijhoff, Dr W. Junk and MTP Press.

Origination by Roby Education Ltd, Liverpool.
Roby Education Ltd., would like to thank the following for their assistance.
Upjohn Ltd.,   Fleming Way, Crawley RH10 2NJ (Joint Aspiration and Injection)
Organon Laboratories Ltd., Milton Road, Cambridge CB4 1BR (Hormone Implant Therapy)
Fern Developments Ltd., 7 Springburn Place, Glasgow G74 5NU (Cryotherapy)

Printed in Gt. Britain by Butler and Tanner Ltd., Frome and London

Contents

Preface

The New Contract which came into force on April 1st 1990 includes proposals for the provision of minor surgery services by the General Practitioner.

The aim of this book is to assist those doctors undertaking minor surgery in their Practices. It is intended to present a practical, clear and concise text. This is accompanied by easy to follow illustrations. The contents of the book are governed by two considerations. Firstly, it covers only those procedures which are safe for the patient. Secondly, it only includes minor surgery which it is possible for the ordinary General Practitioner in a busy practice to undertake.

Chapter One

The Advantages of Minor Surgery in General Practice

Minor Surgery:- Despite this descriptive term, no surgery can be considered "minor" no matter where it is carried out! It requires a knowledge of anatomy and basic surgical principles. There must be an understanding of the procedures and technical skills required. Careful planning is needed at all stages. Arrangements must also be made to deal with any complications and disasters which may occur.

Having stated these provisos, however, surgical procedures can and should be an important part of general practice within the British National Health Service (NHS). There are many advantages to be gained, both for patient and doctor, when minor surgery is undertaken by the general practitioner. The patient is aware of various benefits. The time and travel involved in attending the local hospital will be saved. There should be no prolonged delays in awaiting treatment. It is now taken for granted that, given the present situation and circumstances in the NHS, it can be at least three months before a minor surgical procedure is carried out at a local NHS District General Hospital. This is from the time that the patient is referred by the general practitioner. In contrast, this time scale should be only one or two weeks in general practice.

The familiar surroundings will also be reassuring to the patient, who will appreciate the fact that the surgical operation can be performed by his or her own doctor, or one of the partners in the practice whom he or she knows.

The assistants, nurse and receptionist will also be well known. At the same time there are advantages to the doctor. The general practitioner will be encouraged to maintain an interest in surgery and to practice and continue skills derived from past training. There is also considerable job satisfaction, and bonds between doctor and patient are strengthened. It increases local respect and reputation. Local surgeons will also appreciate many benefits. They will be saved from a workload that can be carried out by general practitioners. The opportunity will be offered for closer professional and personal relations and collaboration between surgeons and their general practitioner colleagues. The development of a local minor surgical service in general practice should be of concern and interest to hospital specialists. They should be consulted and involved in its creation and development and in providing training, advice and back-up for general practice. Ideally, there should be a joint group of surgeons and general practitioners who would plan and promote minor surgery in general practice. They would have responsibility for standards, resources and equipment. Regular exchange visits between surgeons and general practitioners could be arranged. These would involve surgeons being invited to operate occasionally in general practice units to demonstrate techniques. General practitioners would also visit hospital surgical and accident-emergency departments to observe and note facilities and modern equipment.

There should be a benefit to the NHS because it is likely that costs will be saved through fewer referrals to hospital, but this is by no means proven. It may be that such expenses will be merely transferred to general practice.

If, however, there is to be a serious encouragement to general practitioners to undertake minor surgery that is of high standards, then attention has to be given to a system of reimbursement that is much more appropriate than that proposed in the New Contract. Whilst the case for minor surgery is strong, nevertheless there have to be recognized and accepted limits as to what can be carried out safely and successfully.

As will be evident, we believe that practitioners should not undertake any procedures that carry even remote surgical risks to the patient. There should be local protocols agreed between surgeons and general practitioners on what can or should not be carried out in general practice.

Some general practitioners are more skilled surgically because of past experience and may feel able to perform 'hospital' type operations, but nevertheless even they should abide by local rules. The prime consideration has to be the quality of care that the patient receives and it is not surprising that the Royal College of Surgeons is concerned over standards of 'minor surgery' in general practice. Assessment and supervision of these standards must be arranged locally. Medical defence organisations also are concerned that the procedures undertaken by general practitioners will be carried out without increasing risks of disasters resulting in compensation and litigation. No general practitioner should undertake any 'minor' surgery unless he or she has had experience as a junior surgeon in hospital. No GP-surgeon will wish to get into serious difficulties on the practice premises while carrying out 'minor' procedures. Ideally the general practitioner should establish a personal, informal association with a local surgeon and take part in some surgical work at the hospital to maintain his or her skills. The surgeon should also be invited to visit the practice premises, if possible, in order to advise on arrangements and be available if advice or assistance is required.

Although most general practice minor surgery will be carried out in general practice premises, under suitable conditions and with adequate resources (see pages 7-14) there are no reasons why general practitioners should not be given privileges to use local NHS or private hospital facilities, providing that legal and other matters can be agreed.

It is not necessary or even desirable for all general practitioners to become GP-surgeons. It is reasonable that one or more partners in a group practice will undertake all or most of the surgical procedures in special surgical sessions, with 'lists' of collected cases.

The Advantages of Minor Surgery in General Practice

For the patient

- a saving of waiting and travel time
- an enhancement of personal care

For the General Practitioner

- an increase of job satisfaction
- an increase of NHS income
- an increase in status and respect

For local surgeons and hospitals

- less referrals for minor surgery
- promotes better relations with GPs

For the NHS

- a probable reduction in costs and expenditure

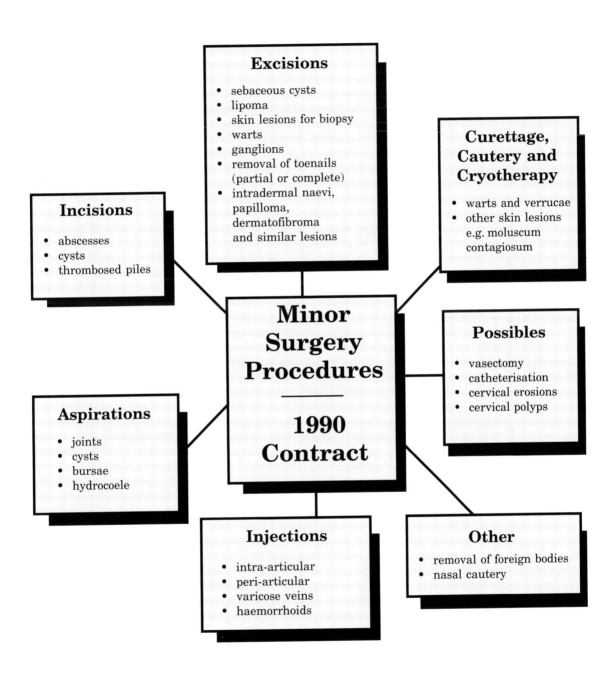

Excisions

- sebaceous cysts
- lipoma
- skin lesions for biopsy
- warts
- ganglions
- removal of toenails (partial or complete)
- intradermal naevi, papilloma, dermatofibroma and similar lesions

Curettage, Cautery and Cryotherapy

- warts and verrucae
- other skin lesions e.g. moluscum contagiosum

Incisions

- abscesses
- cysts
- thrombosed piles

Minor Surgery Procedures

1990 Contract

Possibles

- vasectomy
- catheterisation
- cervical erosions
- cervical polyps

Aspirations

- joints
- cysts
- bursae
- hydrocoele

Injections

- intra-articular
- peri-articular
- varicose veins
- haemorrhoids

Other

- removal of foreign bodies
- nasal cautery

Protocol in General Practice

- only undertake minor surgery which can be performed safely and efficiently

- liaise closely with local surgeons for retraining

- confine procedures to those encouraged under the 1990 contract

Chapter Two

Resources

Good organisation with adequate resources and facilities is required if quality and high standards in minor surgery are to be maintained. There is need for constant regular performance and support and assistance. The occasional ad hoc operator is a potential danger.

Organisation should include arrangements for a suitable place to operate, adequate time and suitable assistance. If possible, a regular 'list' of operations should be drawn up on a set day, at a time outside the normal hurly-burly of general practice. It is essential that there should be no disturbance during this time.

An adequate sized room has to be available with space for work and storage. An operating table or couch should be placed centrally, to allow room for the operator and assistant on either side of the table and at its head. Also required will be a seat for the operator, an arm board for the table or couch, dressing trolleys and a sink with elbow taps. There must be adequate storage space for instrument sets, dressing packs, sutures, lotions, anaesthetics, needles, syringes, containers for disposable waste - including sharps, specimen containers, pillows, sheets and clothing. For each operative session there should be adequate resuscitation equipment, including a minimum of airways of various sizes and staff trained in basic resuscitation procedures. A changing room with access to toilet facilities will also be needed.

Sterile equipment has to be provided and this needs careful preparation. A practice autoclave may be required. This must be checked periodically to assess its effectiveness. Arrangements could be made with the local NHS hospital to provide sterile sets of equipment. This would have to be on the understanding that they will be returned clean and complete, ready for resterilisation and recycling.

Lighting must be an important consideration. There has to be overhead lighting without shadowing. This can be provided by good ceiling fluorescent lamps. A good quality freestanding anglepoise type lamp should also be available, particularly for gynaecological and other procedures.

Basic Essentials for High Standards of Minor Surgery in General Practice

- good organization

- adequate equipment

- adequate facilities

- support and assistance

- careful preparation

- meticulous record keeping

Hazard Warnings

- ad hoc operators are potentially dangerous

- attempting general anaesthesia without expert assistance is highly dangerous

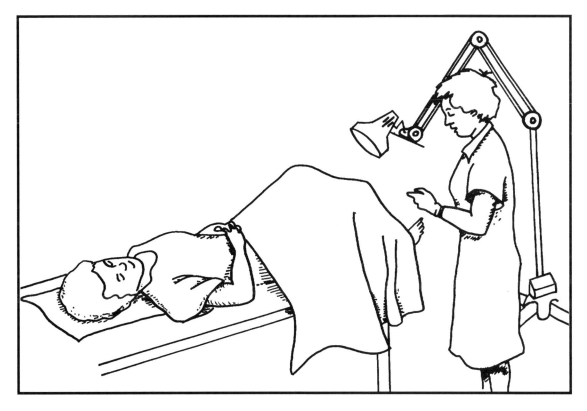

Figure 2.1 A Freestanding Anglepoise Lamp is Recommended

Sterile clothing is not essential provided that the operator and assistants scrub up and use sterile disposable gloves and aprons or gowns.

It is essential to have an assistant present. This is usually the practice nurse, but it may be another colleague. His or her presence will be required at the actual operation for holding instruments and assisting with sutures and ligatures. Further duties required will be to move and adjust lighting, also to help with the preparation of instruments and swabs and their packaging and disposal. Specimens will have to be labelled and despatched with the necessary forms. The presence of an assistant to bring in the patient and provide comfort and reassurance before, during and after the operation, will be of great help. Preparation for the next operation will also need organizing.

The provision of surgical equipment is, to some extent, a matter of personal choice. There has to be, however, a minimum basic set or pack. This must include the following:- scalpels, dissecting scissors, both toothed and non-toothed, two pairs of Allis forceps, plastic trays, swabs and dressings in dry sterile packs. Sutures are also a personal choice, but four to five types should be adequate (See Chapter 3). The choice of local anaesthetic will probably be Xylocaine 1% plain for digits, Xylocaine 1% with adrenaline for other sites. It is important to note possible sensitivity to adrenaline. Marcaine 0.5% is an alternative and is longer acting. General anaesthesia will require special arrangements with a skilled anaesthetist and equipment and should not normally be undertaken.

Basic requirements

- operating table/couch

- seat

- arm board

- dressing trolley(s)

- sink with elbow taps

Storage Requirements

- instruments

- dressing packs

- needles/sutures

- syringes/needles

- local anaesthetic

- specimen containers

- forms/records

- sheets/pillows

- gowns/gloves

Assistant's Role

- assist in operation

- preparation of instruments

- labelling and despatching of specimens

- patient care/support

Surgical Equipment

- scalpels and blades

- dissecting scissors

- Allis forceps

- plastic trays

- dressings

- sutures

Sterilisation Requirements

- practice autoclave

- hospital CSSD supplies

Resuscitation Requirements

- airways

- laryngoscope

- aspirator

- oxygen/set

Local Anaesthetics

- Xylocaine (lignocaine) 1%

- Xylocaine (lignocaine) 1% with adrenaline

- Marcaine 0.5%

Chapter Three

General Principles

To re-emphasize, good minor surgery requires constant practice. The organisation, the resources and the equipment should be the responsibility of one member of the staff. This could be the practice manager, nurse or partner.

When first invited to attend, the patient should be given full information about the operation. Firstly it is necessary to give a clear and simple explanation of what is to be done, the reasons for the operation and a description of the procedure to be followed. It is important to mention any immediate or later after-effects. This information should be repeated, albeit briefly, immediately before operating, either to the patient, or an accompanying relative. The patient should be instructed on what clothes to wear and what to remove before the operation.

Attention should be paid to medico-legal requirements, such as permission to operate, explanation and documentation. An 'operator's book' is essential and should be an accurate record of all procedures carried out. It should indicate when and by whom the minor surgery was carried out with notes on any unusual occurrences. There should also be full notes in the patient's own record envelope.

Before the patient enters the treatment room, there are certain preliminary preparations to be carried out. The minor operating set should be opened and laid out. Swabs, ready for use, should be available, together with cleansing lotions, such as Hibitane or Betadine. Local anaesthetics must already be drawn up in sterile syringes with suitable needles. The table should be prepared with a cover and sheets. Gloves and gowns for the operator must be set out for use.

On entering the room, the patient should be reassured and further explanation given of the steps to be taken. He or she should be placed on the operating table and made comfortable. The lesion which is to be operated on should be exposed and made accessible, with adjustment to the lights to ensure a good field of vision.

The following procedures should be followed in carrying out the operation. Firstly, the area should be towelled up. The skin incision must be planned and marked out on the skin with a fine marking pen or ballpoint. It is important to mark out clearly at this stage because the site of the lesion may be obscured after the injection of local anaesthetic. In general, the incision should be elliptical, and elongation will prevent 'dog-ears' at the wound ends. Local anaesthetic must next be infiltrated all around the lesion ensuring at least 1cm. of numbness. It is then necessary to wait for five to ten minutes to

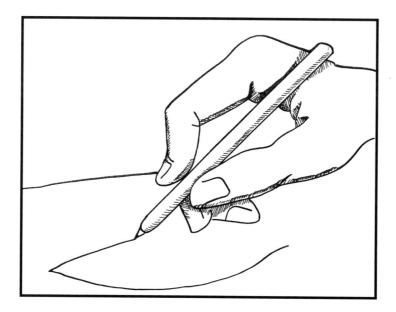

Figure 3.1
Marking Out the
Incision Clearly

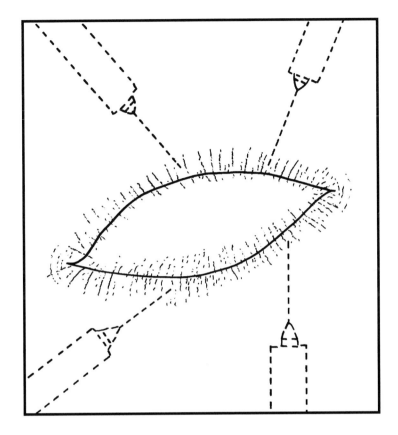

Figure 3.2
Infiltrating All
Around the Lesion

allow the anaesthetic to take effect. During this time, the surgeon and assistant should scrub up. Next, the skin area should be cleansed with Hibitane, or its equivalent, in spirit, or Hibitane in water, or Betadine. Care must be taken during cleansing not to erase the skin marks. An incision should now be made along the line which has been marked out. The scalpel should be held at right angles to the skin, not obliquely, in order to allow good apposition for subsequent suturing. It is necessary to incise through the full thickness of the skin all around the wound, then to free the corners and free the edges from the underlying fat. The edges of large lesions should be undercut with a scalpel to allow them to be brought together before suturing. Large and bleeding vessels should be picked up, clipped and ligated when necessary.

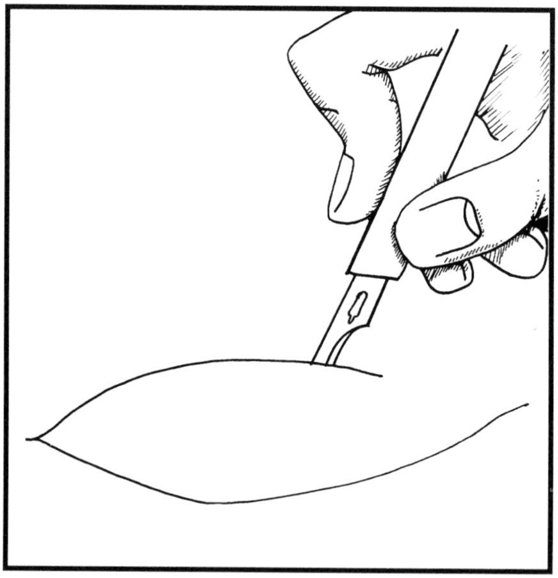

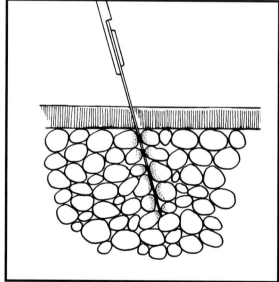

Figure 3.3
Making Elliptical Incision

Figure 3.4
Hold the Scalpel at Right Angles to the
Skin....

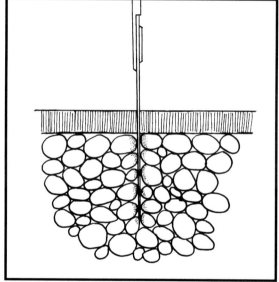

Figure 3.5
.... Not Obliquely.

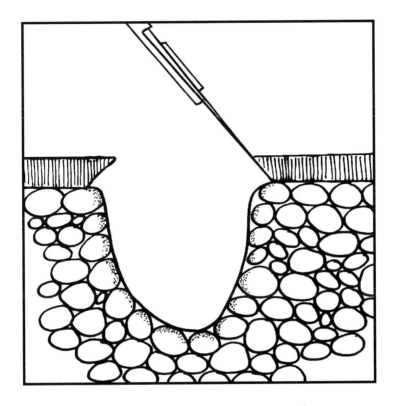

Figure 3.6
Undercutting the
Edges of a Large
Lesion

Suturing should commence at the midpoints of each skin edge. Second stitches should be placed midway between the first stitch and the corners of the wound. The needle holding the suture should pass through the full thickness of the wound edge, across the floor and then up through the full thickness of the other side. The needle should emerge at the same distance from the edges on each side. Mattress sutures will be useful when approximation is difficult. It is important to beware of haematomata occurring due to failed haemostasis, particularly in wounds over concave surfaces. This can be a potent source of infection. In scalp wounds, artery forceps should not be used to control bleeding: large strong sutures, rapidly inserted, will be effective. The use of artery forceps and the ligation of blood vessels to achieve haemostasis will only be necessary where the tissues are lax, or over concave wounds. Catgut should be used in these situations.

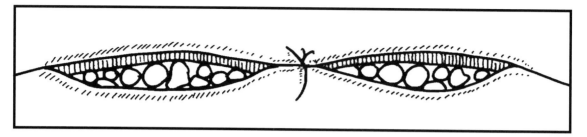

Figure 3.7 Suturing Should Commence at the Midpoints of Each Skin Edge

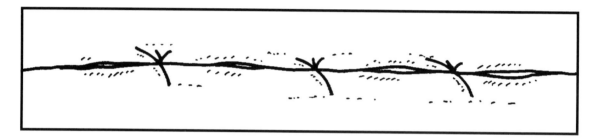

Figure 3.8 Second Stitches

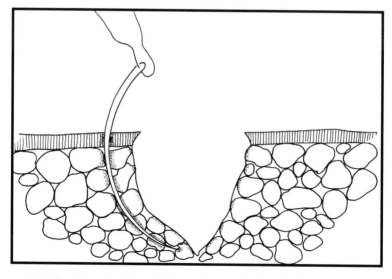

Figure 3.9 The Needle Should Pass Through the Full Thickness of the
Wound Edge and Across the Wound Floor

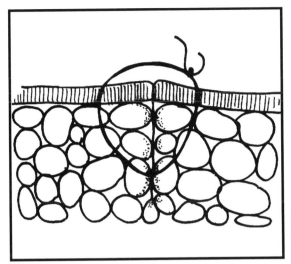

Figure 3.10
The Needle Should Emerge at the Same
Distance from the Edges on Each Side

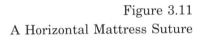

Figure 3.11
A Horizontal Mattress Suture

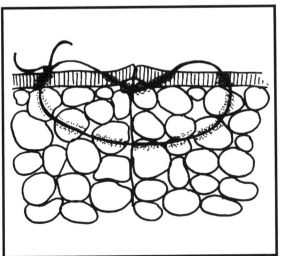

Figure 3.12
A Vertical Mattress Suture

There are various suture materials, such as nylon, prolene, silk, catgut, 'Dexon', etc. Nylon or prolene produce less tissue reaction but they are more difficult to tie and therefore more knots are required. Silk is easier to use but will cause more tissue reaction. Catgut is easy to use and does not have to be removed. It does, however, produce more tissue reactions. It is useful for surgical procedures involving the scrotum and the perineum. 'Dexon' sutures are absorbed only slowly and may have to be removed.

Sutures should not be left in longer than necessary in order to avoid permanent scars. Tissues in the face, scalp, neck, hands and feet heal quickly and sutures can be removed from incisions in these areas in five days, unless there is tension in the wound. Sutures at the front of the neck can be removed even earlier, possibly in three to four days. Incisions in the back and the shin heal more slowly and there is more stretching of the tissues. Sutures have, therefore, to be left in longer, from ten to fourteen days. Sutures in the front of the chest and in the abdomen should be removed after seven days.

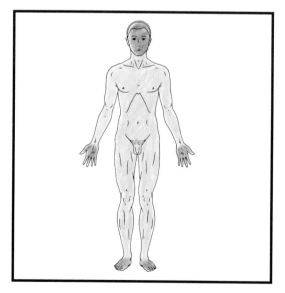

Figure 3.13 Remove Sutures after 5 Days

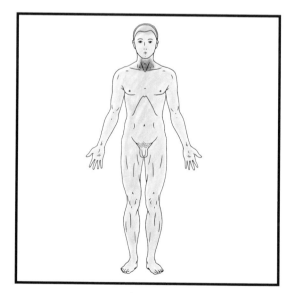

Figure 3.14 Remove Sutures after 3 to 4 Days

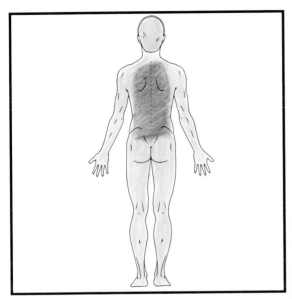

Figure 3.15 Remove Sutures after
10 to 14 Days

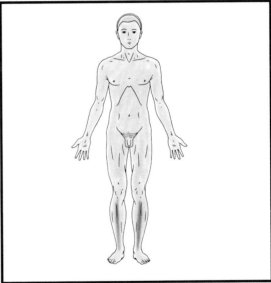

Figure 3.16 Remove Sutures after
10 to 14 Days

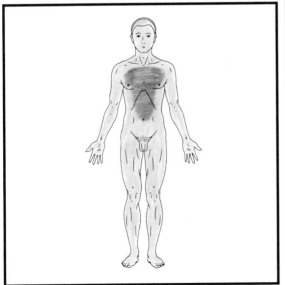

Figure 3.17 Remove Sutures after 7 Days

Dressings will vary according to the situation of the wound. On the face and scalp no dressings are needed. Elswhere, dry gauze should be all that is required. Adhesive tapes or plasters can be used, provided that there is no history of allergy. A proprietary brand, such as Micropore, is probably the safest. It is necessary to keep the wound dry and avoid washing for 24 hours only.

After the operation, it is important to instruct the patient on post-operative care and also to inform him or her of any likely symptoms which may be experienced. Pain should not be a problem and any discomfort should be controllable with simple analgesics, such as paracetamol or co-proxamol. Increasing or severe pain suggests the presence of bleeding and haematoma formation or infection occurring in the wound. In this case the wound needs to be inspected and remedial treatment undertaken if necessary.

All tissues removed should, ideally, be examined histologically both for clinical and medico-legal reasons. Unfortunately, an apparently simple lesion occasionally is found to be malignant. This will then require further specialized investigation and treatment, as a matter of some urgency. Arrangements for these services must be negotiated with local pathologists and surgeons concerned.

Patient's Information

- give clear and simple explanations of procedure

- make known possible after-effects

- advise on clothing to remove and/or retain

Self Protection

- meticulously adhere to medico-legal requirements

- keep clear accurate records in operations book

Post-operative Procedure

- advise patient of post-operative care

- arrange histological examination of removed tissue

- refer all malignancies for specialised investigation and treatment as a matter of urgency

Preparation for Surgery

- have equipment required to hand

- towel up operative area

- re-explain procedure to patient

Chapter Four

Minor Procedures in General Practice

REMOVAL OF SEBACEOUS CYSTS

Sebaceous cysts are the result of blocked sebaceous glands. The sebaceous material is retained in the gland and causes it to enlarge. Once a cyst has reached a size when it is palpable it is unlikely to resolve naturally. If, however, a secondary infection occurs in the cyst and it is severe enough, it may resolve spontaneously.

The removal of the cysts is indicated because of the twofold problems associated with them:- their unsightly appearance and the fact that they are liable to secondary infection.

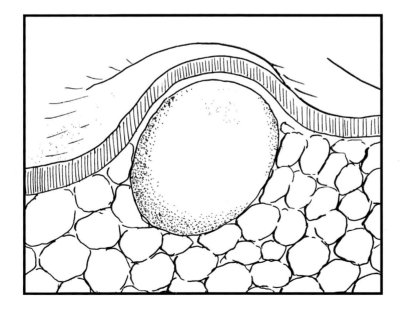

Figure 4.1
Blocked Sebaceous
Gland

The aim of the treatment is to shell out the cyst completely along its line of cleavage. If this is not done successfully it is likely that the cyst will recur.

The following instruments will be required:

- Scalpel

- Dissecting forceps

- Allis forceps

- Needle holder with needle and suture in place

- MacDonald dissector

- Dissecting scissors

- Artery forceps x2

- Dressings, etc.

Firstly it is necessary to mark out the site and the extent of the cyst. Local anaesthetic should be infiltrated around and underneath the cyst. An elliptical incision should then be made. This is deepened until the skin gapes and the cyst or surrounding fat is exposed. The Alliss forceps are then placed on the skin edges so that they may be lifted. The scalpel or dissecting scissors are then used to find the tissue - i.e. the cleavage - plane just around the cyst capsule. The tissue plane is then extended by inserting closed scissor blades into it and separating the handles. Alternatively a scalpel or a Macdonald dissector may be used. If the tissue plane is followed carefully, bleeding should be minimised. An alternative procedure is to cut directly into the cyst, remove the contents, identify the wall and dissect it out completely with scissors.

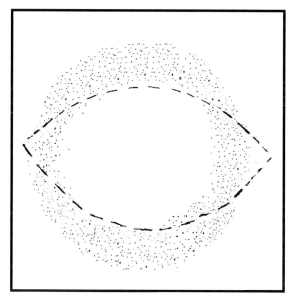

Figure 4.2
Marking Out Site of Cyst

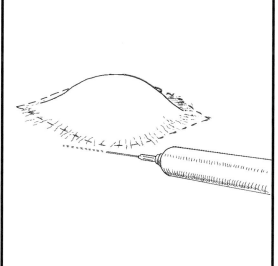

Figure 4.3
Infiltrating with Anaesthetic

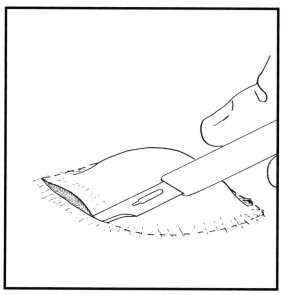

Figure 4.4
Making Elliptical Incision

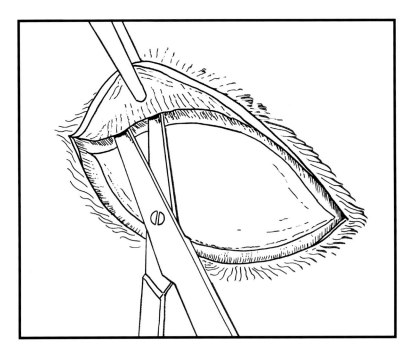

Figure 4.5
Lifting Skin Edges
and Finding the
Tissue Plane

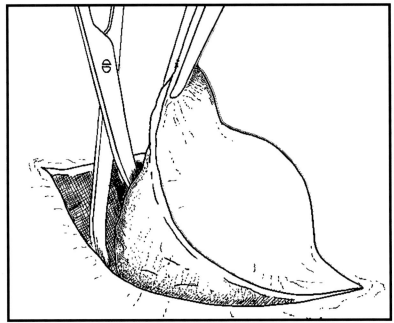

Figure 4.6
Extending the
Tissue Plane

Particular problems may be encountered, depending on the site of the sebaceous cyst. With scalp cysts it is necessary first to shave away the hair from the top of the cyst. During the operation it is advisable to hold a swab below the wound. This will prevent blood trickling through the hair. An even better procedure would be for an assistant to apply pressure to either side of the wound to control bleeding. If all the instruments are ready to hand and sutures are rapidly inserted, bleeding, if any, will be more easily controlled.

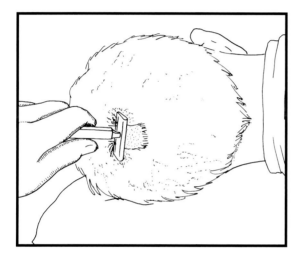

Figure 4.7
Shave Away Hair from
Top of Scalp

Figure 4.8
Incising Cyst and Using Swab to
Prevent Blood Trickling in Hair

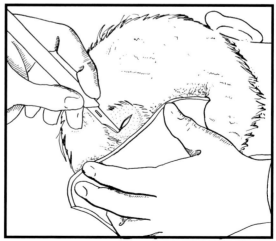

Cysts on the back of the neck also may present problems for the beginner. This is because the skin is tougher in this area. The incision, therefore, has to be much deeper and the dissection is more difficult. Strong sutures may be necessary in the floor of the wound to establish satisfactory haemostasis.

Small cysts occurring on the eyelids are often more easily dealt with by using fine scissors, rather than a scalpel, and then suturing the wound with fine absorbable catgut which does not have to be removed.

There may also be problems if the cysts are infected. The tissue planes will be partly or completely lost. If no obvious capsule is identified, then the contents of the cyst should be evacuated. The base and under edges of the wound must be curetted including all parts of the capsule.

REMOVAL OF LIPOMAS

Lipomas are benign fatty tumours sited in subcutaneous tissue. They are most commonly situated on the back or on the neck, but they can occur anywhere. They may present in all shapes and sizes and their separation from adjacent tissue may vary. Lipomas can be difficult to remove, for there may be no easy planes of separation. This is an especially common problem when they occur on the back of the neck and the back. Many are lobulated with the lobules separated by fibrous bands. The aim of the treatment is to excise the lipoma, leaving a neat scar. Because of the difficulties which may be encountered, excision should only be attempted on smaller lipomas. Larger ones should be referred to hospital. If the incision is incomplete, there will be a recurrence of the problem.

The surgical procedure should be as follows. Firstly, it is necessary to mark out the lipoma on the skin with a skin marker or a ballpoint pen. Next, local anaesthetic should be injected all around the site. With a small lipoma, a linear incision should be made over it. The incision should be deepend until the tumour is seen. The plane of dissection should next be developed in order to enucleate the lipoma. This may prove difficult to carry out. With a larger lipoma an elliptical incision will be required. Larger tumours are usually lobulated. It is necessary to seek the outer edge of a lobule, dissect it out and bring it to the surface with a finger. Adjacent fibrous bands should then be divided with scissors. The whole lipoma should gradually be freed, lifted out and removed.

The resulting wound is often deep and bleeding vessels may require clipping and ligation. Deep sutures will be needed to close the cavity in order to prevent haematoma occurring.

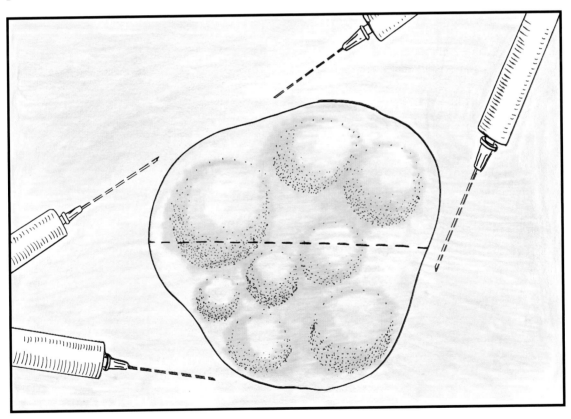

Figure 4.9 Infiltrating Anaesthetic Around the Site

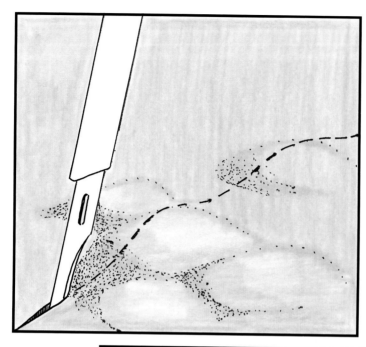

Figure 4.10
Incising Over the
Lipoma

Figure 4.11
Seeking the
Outer Edge of a
Lobule for
Dissection

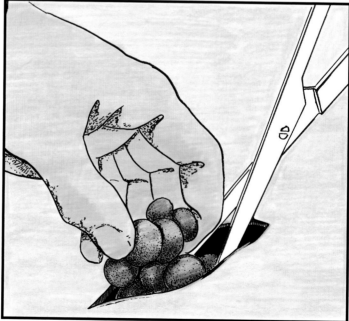

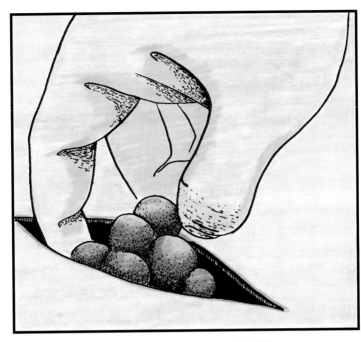

Figure 4.12
Bringing the
Lipoma to the
Surface

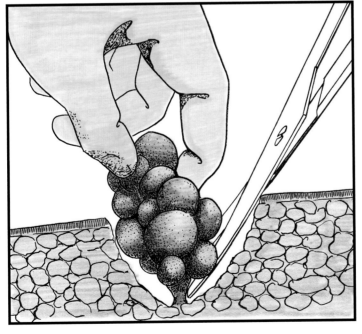

Figure 4.13
Bringing the Whole
Lipoma to the
Surface for Removal

TREATMENT OF TRAUMA AND FOREIGN BODIES

Lacerations and cuts of the skin are universal. There can be few persons who have never had cuts requiring treatment. Depending on the nature of the injury and the object or instrument which caused it, there will be variable amounts of damage to the superficial and deep tissues. Even in apparently surface wounds, it is important to be aware of the possibility of damage to deeper structures.

The aims of the treatment are threefold. Firstly, it is important to achieve as good a cosmetic result as possible; secondly, a good functional result is of great importance; and thirdly, it is necessary to prevent subsequent infection. The treatment involves removing dead tissue, removing any foreign bodies, repairing deeper structures and finally, closing the skin as neatly as possible.

Aims	Effect
• remove dead tissue	
• remove foreign bodies	• good cosmetic result
• repair deeper structures	
• close skin	• good functional result
• prevent infection	

The first step to be taken is to anaesthetise the wound by local infiltration using Xylocaine or Marcaine. The wound should then be cleansed thoroughly with water and explored gently for any foreign material. It is important to check for any damage to deeper structures. It is also necessary to carry out clinical tests to assess any nerve or artery damage. Any dead tissue should then be removed by trimming with scissors.

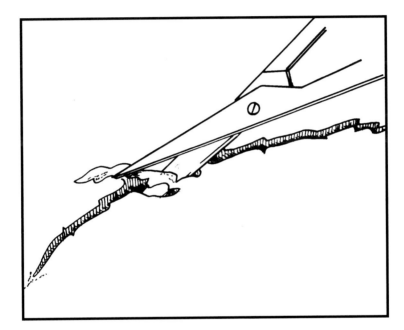

Figure 4.14
Removing Dead
Tissue

Superficial wounds, where the skin edges can be aligned and approximated, can be managed by Steri-Strips. In more difficult injuries, mattress sutures, using nylon, will control bleeding and also result in a good scar. Catgut, however, should be used in deep wounds and where there is damage to the mucosa, as in the mouth. As a general rule, a larger needle is better than a smaller one. Skin sutures may be removed in six to seven days. On the face, however, four to five days is more appropriate. On the back, sutures should remain for a longer period, even up to fourteen days.

Different procedures should be followed, depending on the shape of the wound and its situation. With linear wounds, it is best to start sewing at the mid-points on either side. With V-shaped tears, sewing should start at the apex.

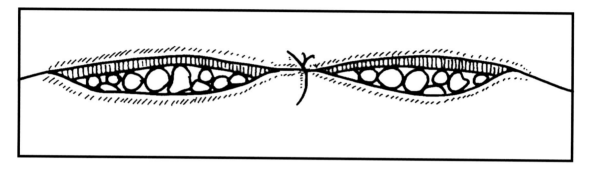

Fugure 4.15 Suturing of Linear Wounds

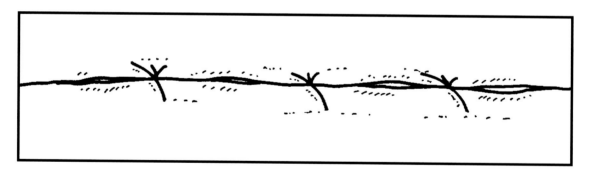

Figure 4.16 Adding Extra Stitches

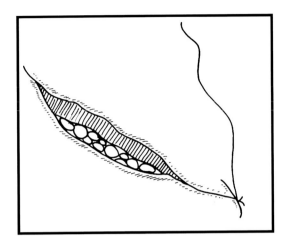

Figure 4.17
Suturing of V-shaped Wound

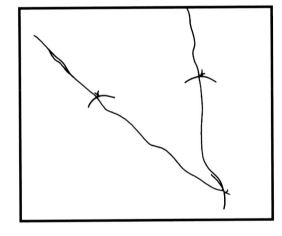

Figure 4.18
Adding Extra Stitches

With cut lips, differing suturing materials will be needed. It is necessary to start sewing edge to edge at the vermilion border with fine nylon sutures. The skin should also be sewn with nylon, but the mucosa must be sutured with catgut.

It is always important to check for tetanus immunisation status. If the last injection was given more than five years previously, then a booster dose of tetanus toxoid (0.5 ml) should be given. In persons with no previous immunisation, a full course should be commenced. If the wound is dirty, it may be advisable to give antibiotics prophylactically. Some form of penicillin would be suitable.

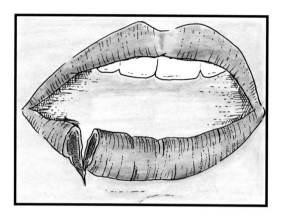

Figure 4.19 Cut Lip

Figure 4.20 Sewing at the Vermilion Border

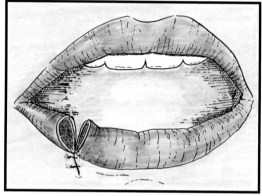

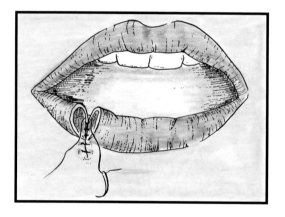

Figure 4.21 Sewing the Mucosa with Catgut

Figure 4.22 Sewing the Skin with Nylon

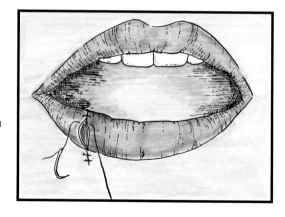

The removal of subcutaneous foreign bodies is usually easy, if the foreign body is palpable. If it is impalpable, however, the patient should be referred to hospital, as X-rays may be required, in order to locate and define the position of the foreign body and facilitate its removal. If the foreign body is palpable, its position should be marked on the surface. Then the area should be anaesthetised by local infiltration or a ring block. An incision should be made directly over the foreign body, which should then be located and removed. In the arm or the leg it is helpful to use a tourniquet; for example, a blood pressure cuff inflated to greater than arterial pressure. Once again a check for tetanus cover must be made.

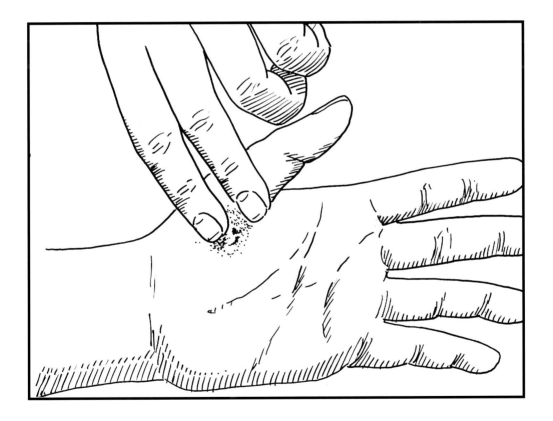

Figure 4.23 Palpating the Foreign Body

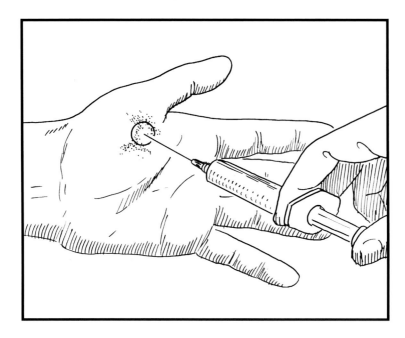

Figure 4.24
Marking the
Foreign Body
and
Anaesthetising
the Area

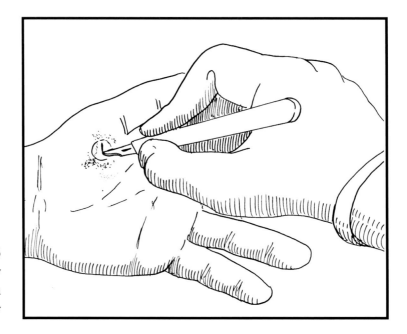

Figure 4.25
Incising Directly
over the Foreign
Body

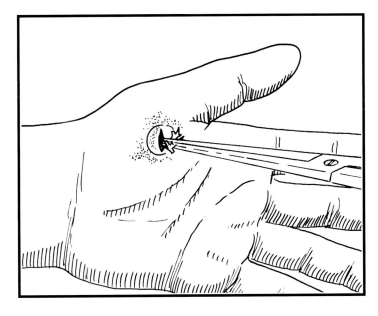

Figure 4.26
Removing the
Foreign Body

MANAGEMENT OF ABSCESSES

An abscess is a localised collection of pus following an infection. The general practitioner undertaking minor surgery will be concerned with abscesses in skin or subcutaneous tissue. Large abscesses, which are deep with overlying induration of the skin, should be treated in hospital. The patient may need to be admitted and the abscess drained under general anaesthetic, possibly with an overnight stay.

A fluctuant abscess suggests that the infection has been localised naturally. If this is the case, the pus can be drained surgically and resolution and recovery will be accelerated. If there is considerable cellulitis and fluctuation is uncertain, it is advisable to treat the patient first with antibiotics. This is particularly so with breast and ischiorectal abscesses. These abscesses tend to be deep and fluctuation can be late or inapparent. If this is the case, they are best dealt with in hospital. It is important to be aware of unusual pathogens and it is wise to send pus for bacteriological tests.

With small or superficial abscesses, it is safe to infiltrate local anaesthetic in and around the centre of the swelling. This can then be incised with a scalpel.

Septic lesions of the fingers and toes require the following considerations. A ring block is the best form of anaesthetic. Deep pulp space infections are now uncommon. They are treated by incisions on either side of the digit, perhaps meeting at the centre. An apical abscess of the pulp is best dealt with by a small incision over the centre of the swelling. Paronychia often requires removal of the nail area as well as incision of the abscess. It is important to maintain function and encourage movements; therefore, dressings should not be restrictive. Persistence of pain after incision suggests that there may have been incomplete drainage. There is also the possibility of underlying bone infection, i.e. osteitis, and further treatment may be required.

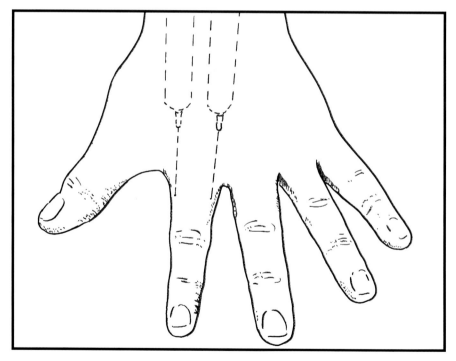

Figure 4.27 Ring Block

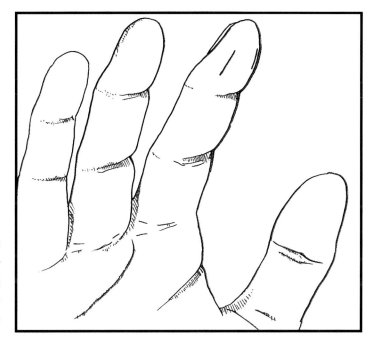

Figure 4.28
Incisions on Either
Side of the Digit
for a Deep Pulp
Space Abscess

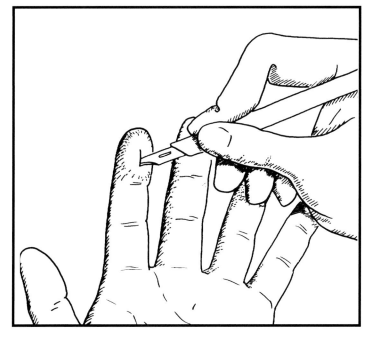

Figure 4.29
Incising an Apical
Abscess

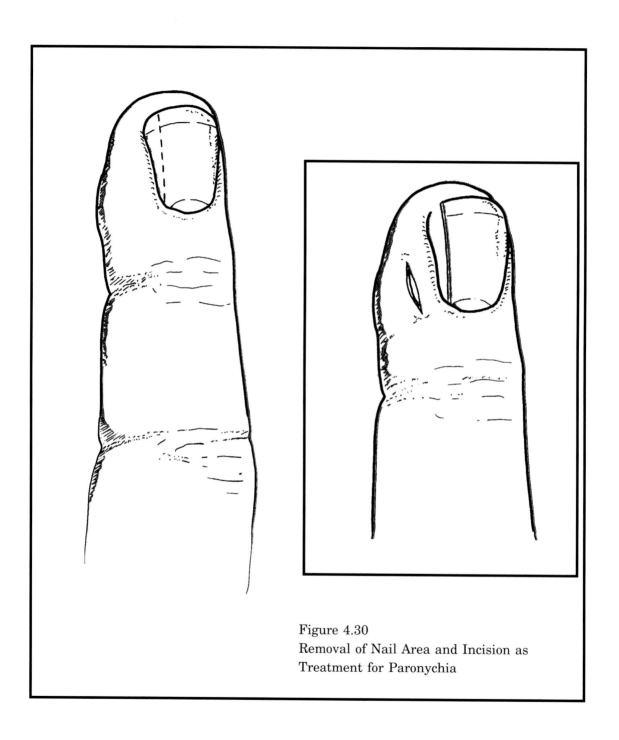

Figure 4.30
Removal of Nail Area and Incision as
Treatment for Paronychia

BREAST CYSTS

Breast cysts are almost always benign retention cysts. They are usually the result of some hormonal dysplastic processes. They are most frequently found in younger women, between the ages of thirty and fifty and are often recurrent. They tend to present as a 'breast lump' that is round, smooth, mobile and frequently tender. Deeper cysts, however, may not be smooth or mobile.

The aim of the treatment is to aspirate the cyst and reassure the patient. Surgical excision is required if the aspirated fluid is bloody or if the cyst does not disappear after aspiration.

The surgical procedure should be as follows. Firstly, a 10 ml syringe should be prepared with a medium or large needle. The cyst must be steadied with the left hand (if the operator is right-handed), and the needle should then be

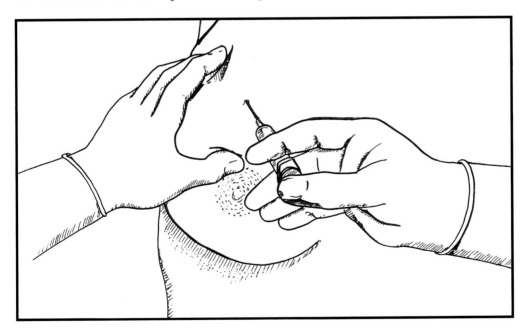

Figure 4.31 Aspirating a Breast Cyst

inserted over the centre of the swelling in order to penetrate the cyst. If the swelling is cystic, there will often be loss of resistance as it is entered. The cyst should then be aspirated completely and the needle withdrawn. The fluid withdrawn may be pale straw coloured, yellow, grey or black and it is not necessary to send it for pathological examination. The swelling should then have disappeared and the patient can be reassured. If, however, the swelling does not disappear, or the fluid is bloodstained, or both, then the patient should be referred to a surgeon. If the diagnosis of 'cyst' has been wrong and the lump is solid, no harm ensues; but referral to a surgeon is again necessary.

CRYOTHERAPY

Cryotherapy is a method of removing warts and other skin blemishes such as spider naevi by freezing with liquid nitrogen or a cryoprobe if one is available.

Firstly, a supply of liquid nitrogen should be obtained. It is best if an arrangement is made with the local hospital dispensary, or with Cryoservice Ltd. Worcester. 'Cotton buds' or orange sticks with cotton wool wound onto the end of the stick should be used for the application. The cotton wool

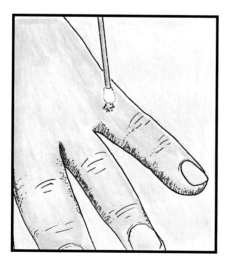

Figure 4.32
Applying Liquid Nitrogen to Wart

should be dipped into the liquid nitrogen and applied to the wart until blanching occurs. The treatment is suitable for hand warts. It is important to take care with warts on extensor surfaces of digital joints, since freezing the joint capsule may occur and cause fibrosis and stiffness.

TREATMENT OF VERRUCAS (PLANTAR WARTS)

Verrucas are warts which are caused by a virus and occur on the soles of the feet and toes. Because of their location, the warts are flattened and pushed into the skin, causing pain. The term 'verruca' causes anxiety to parents, teachers and swimming pool attendants and there is usually pressure to provide treatment. Most verrucas will disappear without treatment, if given time. Local applications are not very successful.

Multiple warts are best treated by cryotherapy. This involves the application of liquid nitrogen or the use of a cryoprobe. Liquid nitrogen is available from the hospital pharmarcy by arrangement, or from Cryoservice Ltd. (Worcester), as noted earlier. The hard skin on the bud should first be shaved with a nail

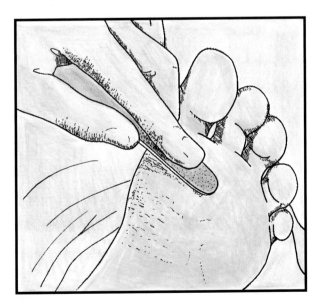

Figure 4.33
Shaving the Verruca
with a Nail File

file. Then the liquid nitrogen should be applied until the skin whitens. If a cryoprobe is available, the same procedure should be followed.

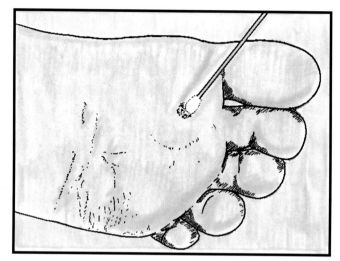

Fugure 4.34
Applying Liquid Nitrogen
to Verruca

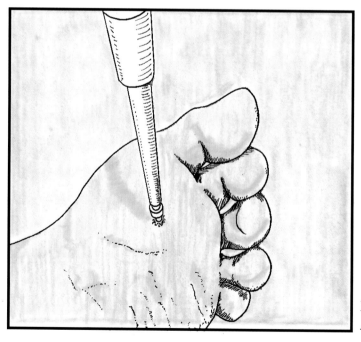

Figure 4.35
Applying Cryoprobe to Verruca

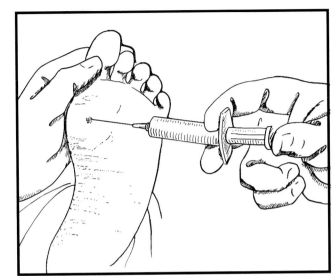

Figure 4.36
Injecting Local Anaesthetic

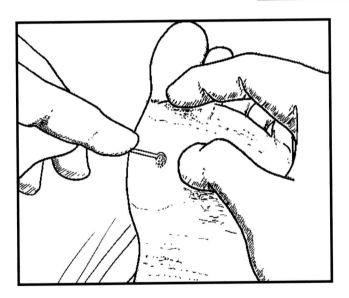

Figure 4.37
Removing Verruca with Curette

Large, horny and solitary warts can be treated by curettage. Local Anaesthetic should first be injected, although this can be very painful. Then the wart should be removed with a curette. After curettage, cautery or trichloracetic acid can be applied, although this is probably unnecessary.

SPECIFIC SKIN BIOPSIES

A specific skin biopsy is indicated when the general practitioner needs a histological examination of a lesion by a histopathologist. It is particularly helpful for skin lumps of doubtful significance and diagnosis. The resulting report may indicate that it is necessary to refer the patient to a specialist for further treatment. Biopsy should not be carried out on a pigmented lesion, which could be a melanoma. This type of lesion is best treated by extensive and deep excision in hospital.

The surgical procedure should be as follows. Firstly , a small area over the lump should be infiltrated with Xylocaine 1% or Marcaine 0.5%. Next a small ellipse of tissue should be excised. The tissue should be placed in a wide-necked container in formol saline solution and despatched to the histopathologist for a report. The wound should be sutured with fine catgut.

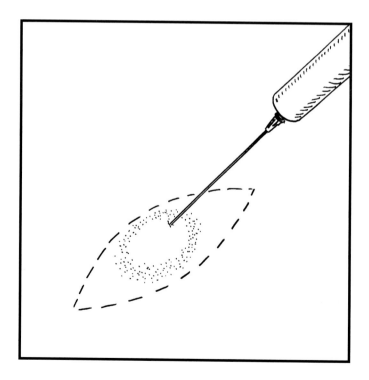

Figure 4.38
Infiltrating in
Preparation
for the Skin Biopsy

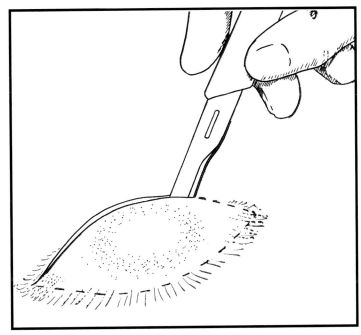

Figure 4.39
Incision for a Skin
Biopsy

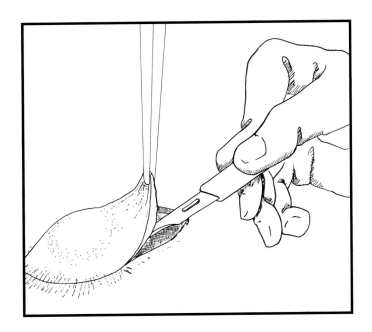

Figure 4.40
Exising Ellipse
of Tissue

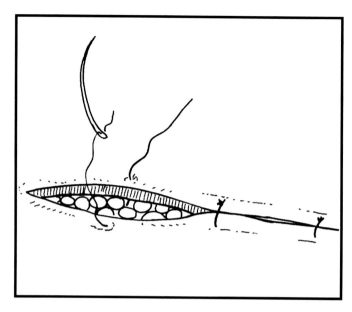

Figure 4.41
Suturing the Wound

MANAGEMENT OF INGROWING TOE NAILS

'Ingrowing toe nails' are not in fact 'ingrown'; that is, they not do grow into the soft tissues. The condition is really a paronychia or a subacute or chronic infection of cutaneous tissue along the sides of the nail of the first toe. It can affect the inner or outer side, or both together. The condition usually follows trauma to the nail edge. This may have been brought about by injudicious cutting of the nail, tightly fitting shoes that cause pressure, or some other form of trauma. Once the infection has started, it tends to persist because the nail edge acts as an irritant. It is difficult to apply local treatment with the nail in situ. Even after an apparently successful treatment, recurrence is likely. The condition is most prevalent in teenagers and affects males more than females.

Resolution is unlikely to occur in a short time unless the nail edge is removed. In chronic or recurrent cases it will be necessary also to excise or ablate the nail bed to prevent the nail regrowing. There are, therefore, two surgical choices. Firstly, the partial removal of the nail edge on the side of the infection: secondly, the removal of the nail, plus the ablation of the nail bed to prevent the nail from regrowing and becoming reinfected. A similar procedure is indicated for onychogryphosis.

The patient should be given a full and honest explanation of the treatment. This should set out the aims of the operation, the steps to be undertaken, the follow up and outcome and also the chances of recurrence.

Anaesthesia has to be effective as the procedure is quite painful. Local ring block is the best method. 10 mls. of plain Xylocaine 1% or plain Marcain 0.5% should be drawn up into a sterile syringe with a fine needle attached.

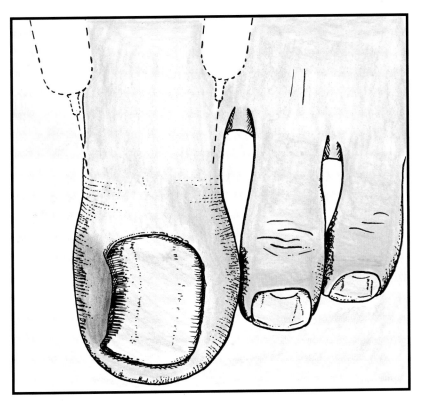

Figure 4.42 Local Ring Block

3-4 mls. of the solution should then be injected on either side of the first proximal phalanx. The needle is moved along the line of the injection site, close to the bone, and the solution is infiltrated in all directions. It is important to wait at least five minutes to allow for complete anaesthesia.

Once the digit is completely numb, the operation area should be cleaned and draped. If an ablative procedure is to be carried out, then a rubber tube tourniquet is placed around the base of the toe with a first throw of a knot and tightened; this may be kept in place with an artery forceps close to the knot.

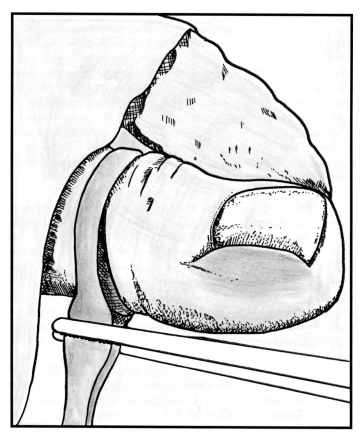

Figure 4.43 Applying Tourniquet to Base of Toe

For the partial removal of the nail, one blade of a pair of scissors, or a MacDonald dissector, should be passed and the nail edge cut away and removed. When partial ablation of the nail bed is indicated, the incision must be carried down to expose the whole of the corner of the base of the nail bed, so that it can be excised. Flaps of skin should be turned back and the nail bed removed. Deep sutures should be used to repair the wound and appose the wound edges and control any bleeding.

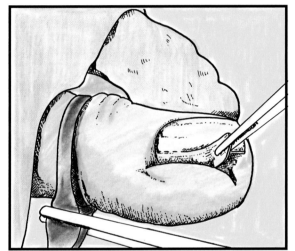

Figure 4.44
Removal of Nail Edge

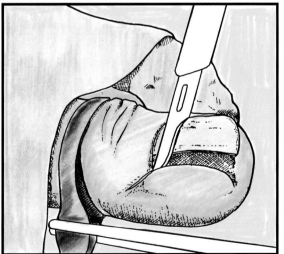

Figure 4.45
Exposing Corner of Nail Bed

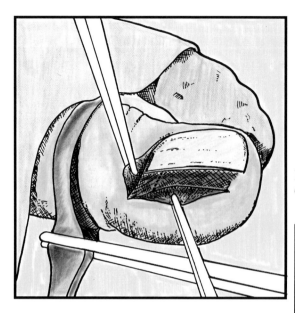

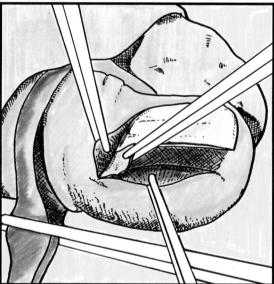

Figure 4.46
Turning Back the Flaps of Skin

Figure 4.47
Removal of the Nail Bed

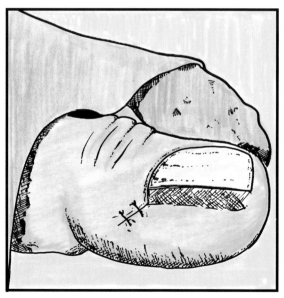

Figure 4.48
Repairing Wound with Deep Sutures

The total ablation of the nail bed involves removal of the whole germinal matrix. This must be excised after extensive reflection of the skin flap. It is important to remove the complete nail bed into the corners to prevent small spikes of new nail from regrowing. The nail fold should then be advanced and sutured. A single layer of tulle gras should be applied to the wound and then a layer of gauze, which can be kept in place by Elastoplast. Alternatively, Tubegauze can be applied.

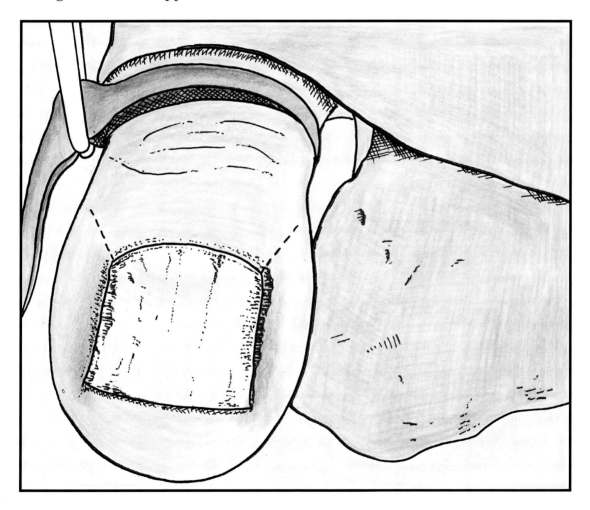

Figure 4.49 Incisions for Zadek's Operation

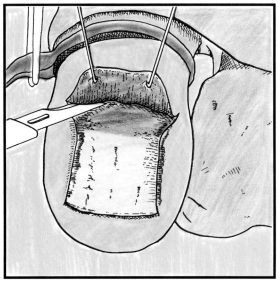

Figure 4.50
Reflection of the Skin Flaps

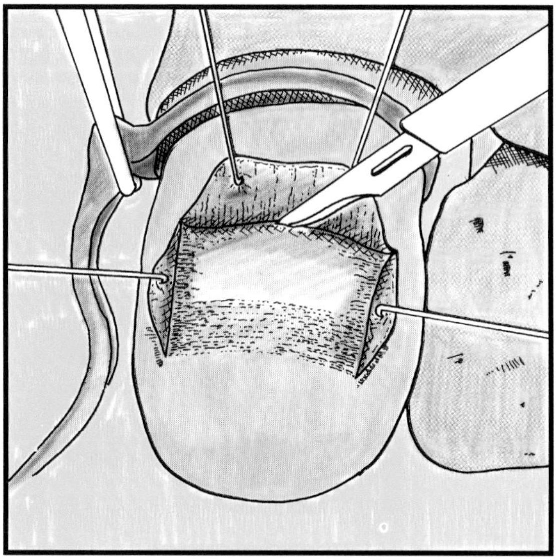

Figure 4.51
Nail Removed and Releasing of the Nail Bed

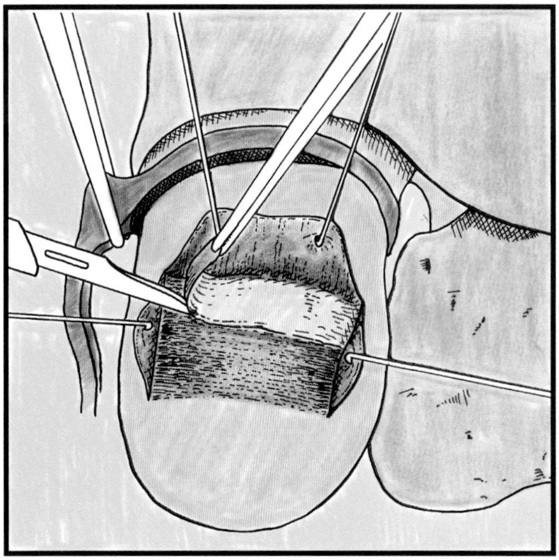

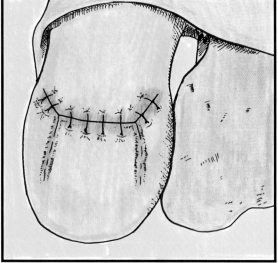

Figure 4.52
Removal of Nail Bed

Figure 4.53
Suturing of Nail Fold

The patient should remain on the couch for five to ten minutes. The wound must then be inspected to ensure no further bleeding has occurred. The patient should return next day when the bulky dressing can be removed and be replaced by a smaller dressing. Sutures may be removed in three to four days. Healing is usually rapid.

TREATMENT OF PERIANAL HAEMATOMA

Perianal haematoma is an acute painful swelling in the subcutaneous tissues at the edge of the anus. It is caused by the rupture of a small subcutaneous perianal vein which produces a small clotted haematoma. Patients usually come complaining of 'piles'. The first step must be to establish the diagnosis and reassure the patient. Spontaneous resolution usually occurs in seven to fourteen days. If there is only a little pain or discomfort, then it is advisable to allow the natural resolution of the haematoma to occur and strongly reassure the patient that this will happen. If the haematoma is very painful it should be incised and expressed.

It is necessary to discuss the management of the condition with the patient and explain the procedure to be followed. If the patient agrees to the removal of the haematoma then the following steps should be taken. Firstly it is necessary to anaesthetise the area around the swelling with a local injection

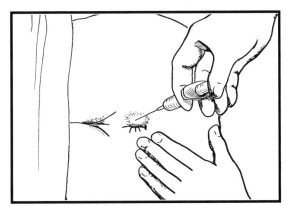

Figure 4.54
Anaesthetising the Area
Around the Swelling

of Xylocaine or Marcaine. Then the swelling should be incised and the haematoma expressed digitally. This should provide instant relief and no sutures are required. Bleeding may occur from the incision and is best controlled by local pressure. It is important to beware of misdiagnosing prolapsed piles, because incision of these will cause very severe bleeding.

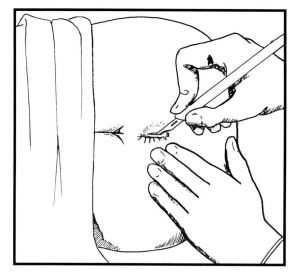

Figure 4.55
Incising the Swelling

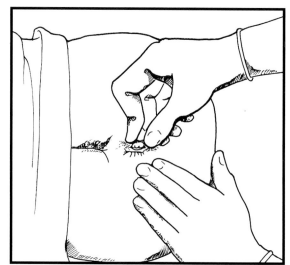

Figure 4.56
Expressing the Haematoma

INJECTION OF PILES

Piles are vascular ano-rectal 'cushions' that become congested and enlarged. Three grades are recognized. The first is bleeding only; the second is bleeding with prolapse only at defecation; the third degree stage is bleeding with prolapse at defecation and also at other times. At this stage, it is also necessary for the patient to replace the prolapsed piles.

As noted, perianal haematomata are not piles. Rectal bleeding is not always caused by piles. More serious causes must be excluded before any treatment is commenced. Ideally, therefore, anyone being treated for anorectal conditions should have a sigmoidoscopy to exclude cancer of the rectum. Any suspicious lesions, such as polyps or tumours, must be biopsied and specimens sent for histological examination. The mucosa in proctitis should also be sent for histology. Proctoscopy is insufficient as many lesions occur beyond the length of the proctoscope.

The first step to be taken in treating a person with rectal bleeding is to make certain that it is not due to cancerous lesions in the rectum or the colon. Many persons have occasional solitary rectal bleeds, which may be due to piles and which may cease without treatment. The bleeding may also cease if a faulty diet is corrected. First degree piles and some second degree piles can be treated with sclerosing injections. Ideally, sigmoidoscopy should be carried out before treating bleeding piles. If, however, there are no clinical pointers to other gastrointestinal pathologies and if rectal examination is normal, then the procedure is justifiable without sigmoidoscopy, providing adequate follow-up is ensured.

The following equipment is required. There must be a good source of light; an anglepoise lamp will suffice. A proctoscope, a haemorrhoid syringe and oily phenol, i.e. phenol in arachis oil, are also needed. Proctoscopes and sigmoidoscopes, with light attachments, syringes and needles, are now available as disposables.

With the patient in a left lateral or knee-elbow position, the proctoscope is inserted and the obturation removed. Slight withdrawal of the proctoscope reveals the projecting piles. 2-3ml. of oily phenol is injected into each of the three pile areas. It is important to take care not to inject phenol into the prostatic substance. Oily phenol is messy and gauze or some other absorbent material should be tucked underneath the buttock. This will absorb any oil on withdrawal of the proctoscope.

If rectal bleeding has been due to piles, then injection rapidly controls it. If bleeding continues, then more investigations are essential. This is particularly important if there are accompanying abdominal symptoms or changes in bowel habits.

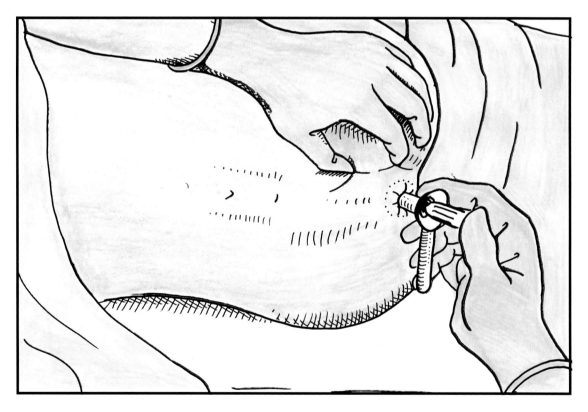

Figure 4.57 Insertion of the Proctoscope

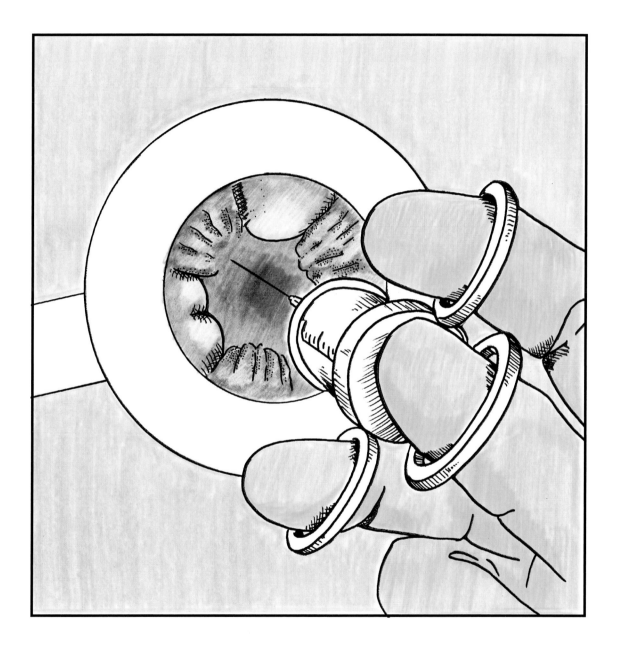

Figure 4.58 Injection into the Pile Areas

INJECTION OF VARICOSE VEINS

Varicose veins arise commonly from venous valve incompetence occurring at valves at the upper end of the long or short saphenous veins, or incompetence of the valves from perforating veins connecting deeper venous systems. Sclerosant injection of varicose veins leading to thrombotic fibrosis is most likely to be successful when there is no sapheno-femoral or short saphenous incompetence. The patient should stand on a stable stool with legs exposed. The presence of a cough impulse in the groin should be noted and any palpable veins there, or in the popliteal area, should also be noted. If these are absent, then sclerotherapy is justifiable.

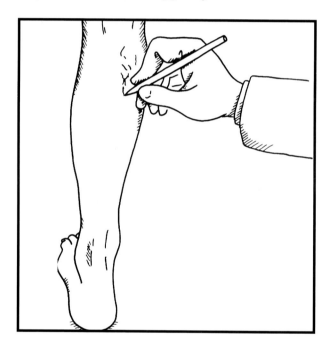

Figure 4.59
Marking Out the
Varicose Veins
with the Patient
Standing

Suitable veins should be marked with a ballpoint pen whilst the patient is standing. Three or four 2ml. syringes should be loaded with 0.5ml. of STD (sodium tetradecyl sulphate). The patient should then lie down. The veins must then be localised and STD injected only when the operator is sure that

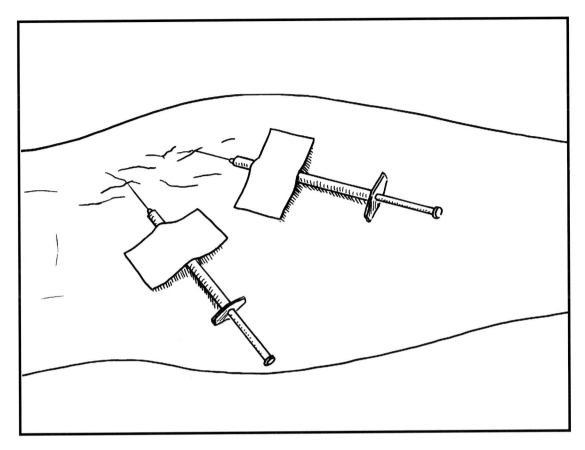

Figure 4.60 Injecting the Varicose Veins with STD

the needle is in the vein. After injection, local pressure is applied with gauze to prevent extravasation of the sclerosant. Pressure is continued for a few days by application of small sponges supported by bandages. The patient should be asked to walk briskly for twenty to thirty seconds after injection to promote local circulation and prevent deep vein thrombosis. The patient should be warned to expect local tender and painful lumps at the sites of the injections. These will take two or three weeks to settle and there may be some residual brown staining of the skin.

LIGATION OF VARICOSE VEINS

This may be a hazardous procedure in the groin region and is not to be recommended. In other situations, clusters of two or three varices can be ligated. Firstly, the veins should be marked out on the skin, with the patient standing as before. Then, after the site of ligation has been decided, the patient should lie down. The skin should be infiltrated with local anaesthetic. Next, incisions should be made across the lines of the veins. Then the incisions should be deepened and the veins defined by blunt dissection. Two artery forceps should then be applied and the veins cut. The ends of the veins should be ligated with 2-0 catgut. If there is bleeding, the leg should be elevated to control it. If the vein walls are thin, dissection may be difficult. In this case, it is necessary to transect the vein and under-run each end with catgut stitch.

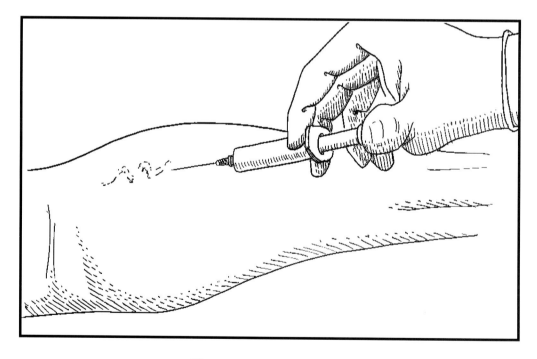

Figure 4.61 Infiltrating the Site of the Varicose Veins

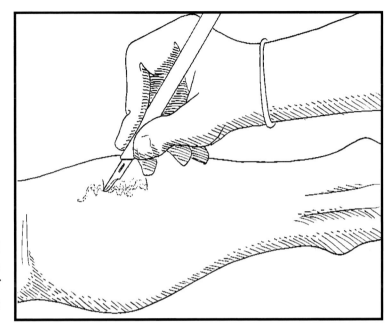

Figure 4.62
Incising Across
the Lines of
the Veins

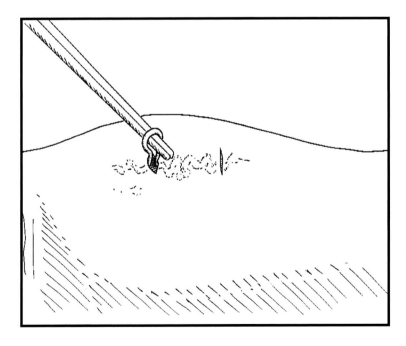

Figure 4.63
Defining the
Veins by Blunt
Dissection

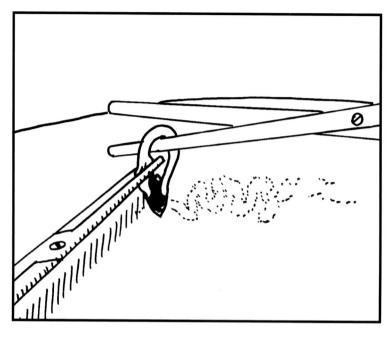

Figure 4.64
Cutting the Veins

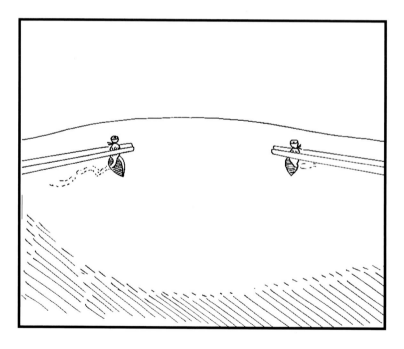

Figure 4.65
Ligating the Veins
with Catgut after
the Removal of
Varicosities

HYDROCOELE TAPPING

A hydrocoele is an encysted collection of fluid within the tunica vaginalis in the scrotum, above and in front of the testis. It occurs most frequently in middle aged and elderly men. It is usually primary, but may be secondary to disease of the testis. Congenital hydrocoele in infants is common and may disappear spontaneously. If it does not disappear, it is usually communicating with the peritoneum and herniotomy is the most usual treatment. The optimum treatment for hydrocoele is surgical operation in hospital, but some patients prefer intermittent tapping to evacuate the fluid. Recurrence is usually to be expected.

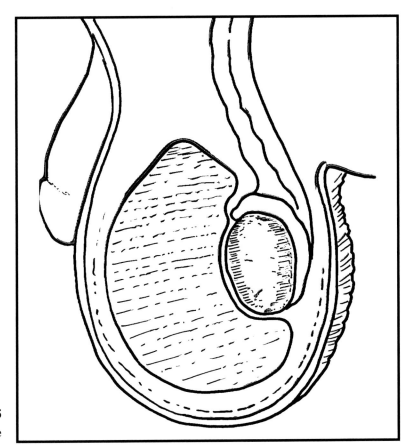

Figure 4.66
Hydrocoele

Tapping a hydrocoele should be a straightforward and safe procedure. Firstly, it is necessary to confirm that the swelling is a hydrocoele. This can be ascertained by 'getting above' the swelling and transilluminating it. It is important not to confuse the condition with a scrotal hernia in an obese elderly man. The testis should be palpated to check that it is normal. In a tense hydrocoele, the testis can only be checked after the removal of the fluid.

The following instruments are required:

- trocar and cannula
- cleansing fluid
- local anaesthetic
- syringe and needle
- scalpel blade
- kidney dish

The patient should lie on the couch with legs apart and trousers and pants removed. The scrotum is then cleaned and a kidney dish placed beneath to collect the fluid. The swelling should be steadied with the left hand and the skin stretched over the hydrocoele. A little anaesthetic should be infiltrated into the skin and the underlying tunica at the chosen site of puncture. A small cut is then made, with the scalpel, to facilitate the penetration of the tissues by the trocar and cannula. The trocar and cannula should then be firmly inserted into the hydrocoele. When the trocar is withdrawn, the clear, yellow fluid can be collected by gentle squeezing of the scrotum. It is important to prevent the cannula from moving out, as it may come outside the tunica and the flow of liquid will cease. Then a complete repetition of the procedure will be necessary in order to insert the cannula back into the hydrocoele. When the hydrocoele has been emptied, it is important to check the testis. Finally, the skin wound should be cleaned and collodion or Actaflem applied to the small wound. Bleeding may occur rarely into the tunica during the procedure. This will cause a painful haematoma within the scrotum, which will take a long time to resolve.

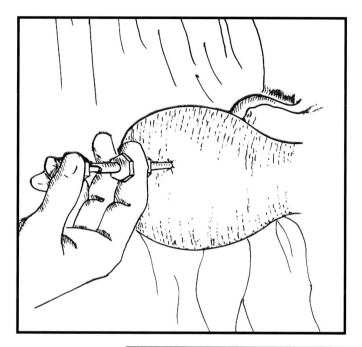

Figure 4.67
Anaesthetising the
Scrotum

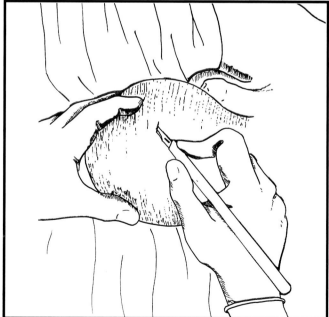

Figure 4.68
Incising the
Scrotum

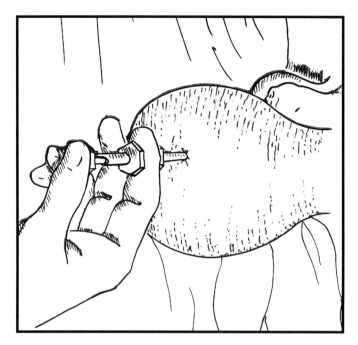

Figure 4.69
Inserting the Trocar
and Cannula

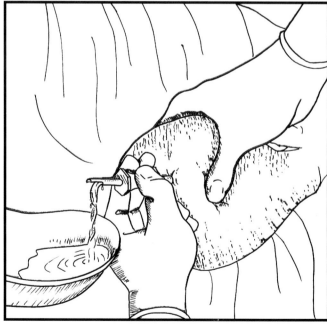

Figure 4.70
Draining the Fluid

Colour Atlas of Minor Surgery in General Practice

CATHETERISATION

The need for catheterisation is indicated when there is acute retention of urine, or when the patient is incontinent. For male catheterisation, a size 16-18 Foley catheter is the basic size. It is advisable to use a larger catheter rather than a smaller one, in order to avoid creating a false passage. The patient should lie with legs apart and trousers and pants removed. The penis should be cleaned with cetrimide. Then Xylocaine gel should be inserted into the urethra for anaesthesia. A penile clamp is then applied for five minutes. During this time, the operator should scrub and towel up the patient. The end of the Foley catheter should be lubricated and inserted into the bladder, after removing the penile clamp. Then the balloon should be inflated with water and drainage commenced if necessary.

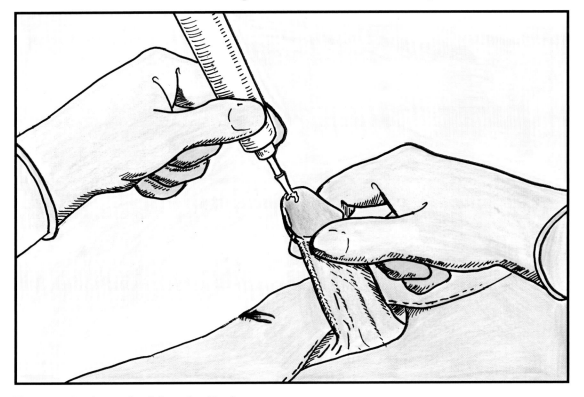

Figure 4.71 Anaesthetising the Penis

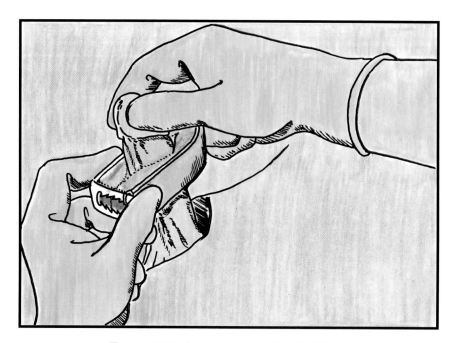

Figure 4.72 Application of Penile Clamp

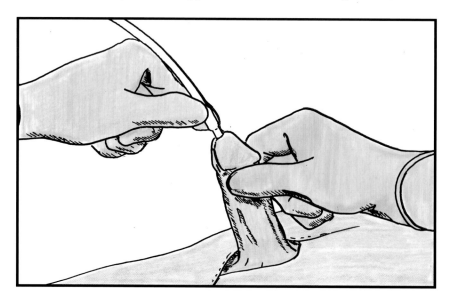

Figure 4.73 Insertion of Catheter into Penis

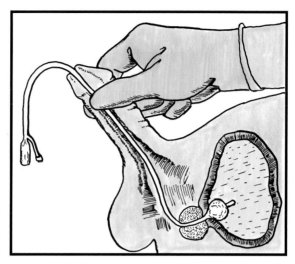

Figure 4.74
Expansion of Balloon in
Preparation for Drainage

In female catheterisation, local anaesthesia is not necessary. The patient should lie with legs apart. The vulva should be cleaned with cetrimide. After visualising the urethral opening, a lubricated Foley catheter should be passed.

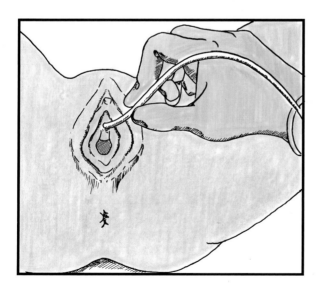

Figure 4.75
Insertion of Catheter into
Urethral Opening

VASECTOMY

Vasectomy is the sterilisation of the male by ligation and division of both vasa deferens at the upper end of the scrotum. It is important always to check that there are no accessory vasa. The aim of the operation is to achieve total aspermia. This must be checked for, by semen analysis, four to six weeks after the operation. There will be medico-legal consequences if sterilisation is incomplete.

In general practice it is assumed that the procedure will be carried out under local anaesthetic, preferably with an assistant , who is also scrubbed up. It is important to make sure that all instruments which may be required are laid out. Everything should be prepared before the patient enters, as he may be both anxious and afraid. It is essential to explain the procedure to be followed and what the patient will feel happening during the operation. The patient should lie in a supine position, with legs apart. The area should have been shaved by the patient with a safety razor. After towelling up, the vas on both sides should be localised by palpation. The vas should then be lifted

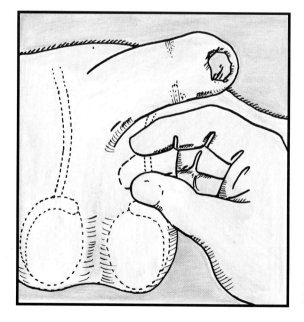

Figure 4.76
Palpatating the Vas

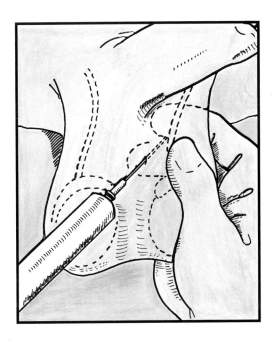

Figure 4.77
Infiltrating Around the Vas

up and stretched over the forefinger; it can be steadied with the help of the assistant at this stage. Local anaesthetic, such as Xylocaine with adrenaline, should then be infiltrated around the vas and the skin over the vas incised. The next step is to locate and define the vas and place an Allis forceps around it. A linear incision must then be made over the top of the vas to expose it and more local anaesthetic injected beneath the loop of vas. One inch of bare vas should then be dissected out and freed. After applying clips, a half to three quarters of an inch should be excised between the clips and the two ends tied with catgut. It is important to check carefully for any bleeding points around the vas or its mesentery. These should be clipped and tied off, as haematoma can be very painful and also liable to infection. The scrotal wound should then be closed with deep catgut sutures, to ensure haemostasis. The skin should be sprayed with a plastic sealant, such as Optaflex, and then covered with small squares of gauze. The procedure is then repeated on the other side. The patient should be informed that there will be soreness for a few days, that the sutures will dissolve and that he can bathe or shower in a few hours.

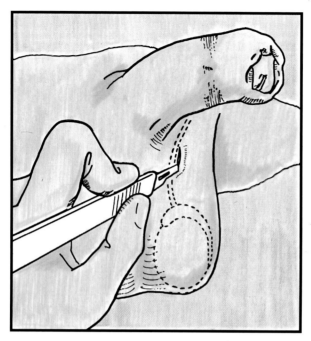

Figure 4.78
Incising Over the Vas

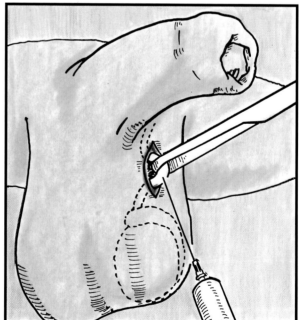

Figure 4.79
Injecting Beneath Vas Loop

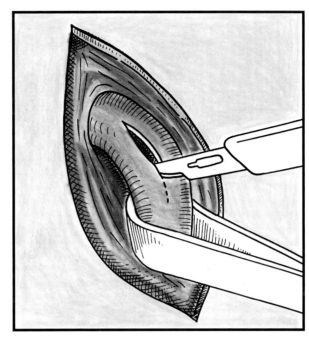

Figure 4.80
Incising Vas Sheath

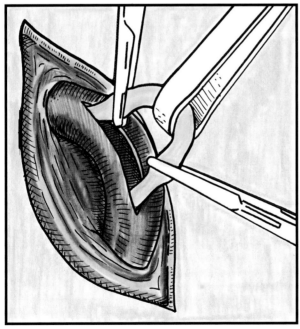

Figure 4.81
Freeing Bare Vas

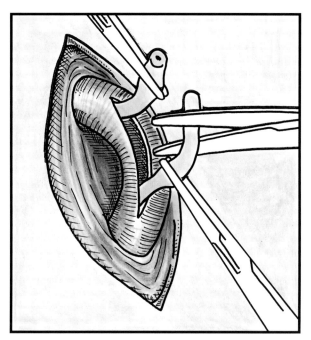

Figure 4.82
Excising Vas

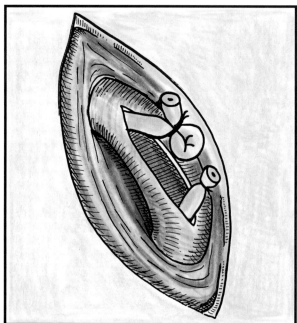

Figure 4.83
Tying Ends with Catgut

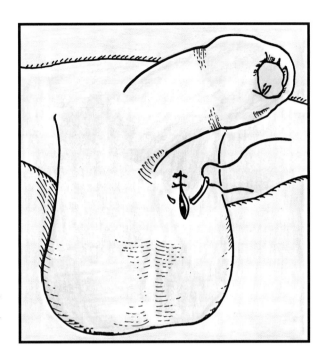

Figure 4.84
Suturing the Scrotum

Chapter Five

Injection and Aspiration of Joints and Soft Tissues

Injection and aspiration of accessible joints and surrounding soft tissues are safe and effective procedures to perform in general practice. They are little different to other forms of injection of vaccine and drugs and to aspiration in the form of venesection. Provided that basic rules of sterility are followed and local anatomy is understood, few problems should be encountered.

There are both therapeutic and diagnostic objectives in using these procedures. The therapeutic aims are to treat local inflammatory reactions by injection of steroid preparations into a joint or infiltration of tissues around it to achieve their anti-inflammatory effects. The process of aspiration of fluid from a joint, ganglion or cyst may itself relieve or cure the condition. The diagnostic aims are to obtain fluid from a joint, which can then be analysed, in order to differentiate between conditions such as gout, infection or simple inflammatory swellings.

It is important to make as accurate a diagnosis as possible. If the condition is one that is likely to respond to local injection of steroid, it is advisable to arrange for this procedure to be carried out. The technique need not be any more complicated or difficult than giving an intramuscular, intravenous or subcutaneous injection. Sterile disposable syringes and needles of various sizes are freely available to NHS general practitioners. Normal aseptic precautions should be taken for the procedure, using the appropriate size needle and syringe.

The most popular preparation in use is Depomedrone (methylprednisolone). Depomedrone is available in vials of 1ml. and 2ml. (40mg. per ml.). It is often used mixed with Xylocaine 2% (lignocaine) for its local anaesthetic effect to reduce local pain. The most important factor for success is to place the injection in the correct site, based on a knowledge of pathology and anatomy. Depending on the site and the tensions of tissues, between 0.5-2ml. of Depomedrone are recommended.

In the following specific situations the use of Depomedrone will be of great value, as will other procedures, such as aspiration, in order to relieve pain and reduce disability.

SHOULDER

The shoulder is often affected by acute and persistent pain and stiffness. Accurate diagnosis can be difficult and often impossible. The most likely diagnoses are generalised capsulitis (frozen shoulder), supraspinatus tendinitis, or acromio-clavicular and sterno-clavicular disorders.

In generalised capsulitis or 'frozen shoulder' there is no discrete localised tenderness but there is painful stiffness in all directions. The condition often

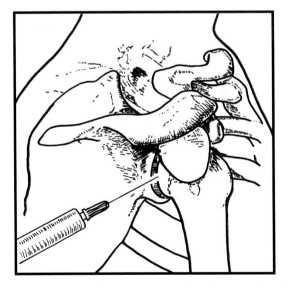 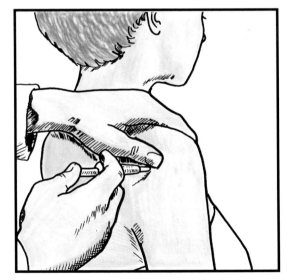

Figure 5.1 and 5.2 Injection for Frozen Shoulder

takes a long time to recover naturally. It may take as long as one to two years. The injection of steroid may be helpful in order to relieve pain and shorten the period of recovery. 2ml. of Depomedrone should be injected into the periarticular tissues at the back of the shoulder, below and medial to the tip of the acromion process.

In supraspinatus tendinitis there is tenderness laterally over the humerus at the sub-acromial area and a painful arc of abduction. The injection of 1-2 ml. of Depomedrone at this site can be dramatically successful.

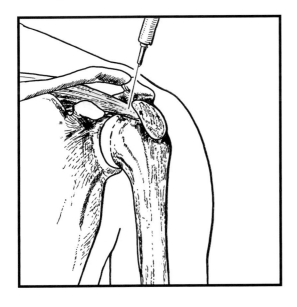

Figure 5.3 and 5.4 Injection for
Supraspinatus Tendinitis

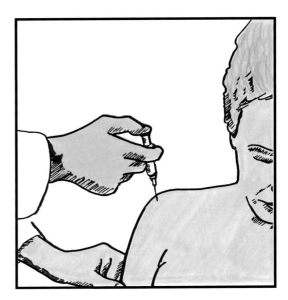

Acromio-clavicular and sterno-clavicular tenderness, especially following injury, such as falls, respond well to the injection of 1ml. of Depomedrone.

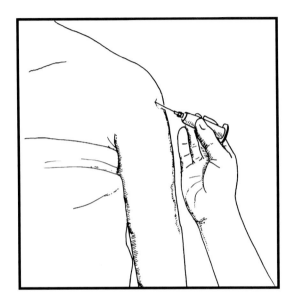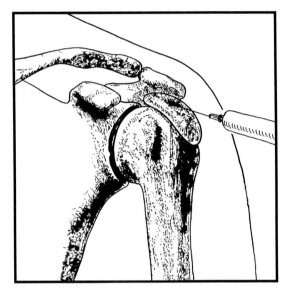

Figure 5.5 and 5.6 Injection for Acromio-Clavicular Tenderness

ELBOW

There are various conditions which cause pain in the elbow. In 'tennis elbow', lateral epicondylitis, the classical symptoms are pain on gripping, e.g. when shaking hands, and lifting, e.g. using a teapot, or carrying bags. There is also exquisite tenderness on palpation. The injection of Depomedrone 0.5-1ml., with or without Xylocaine, into the most tender site and around it is the most effective treatment, but it does not always succeed and recurrence is common. It is always important to warn the patient that pain is often worse for one to two days after the injection.

'Golfers elbow' is medial epicondylitis and the treatment is similar to that of 'tennis elbow'.

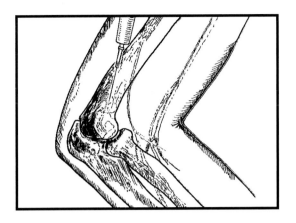

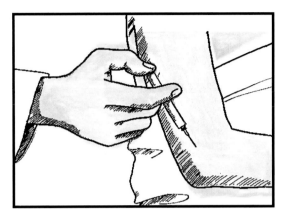

Figure 5.7 and 5.8 Injection for Tennis Elbow

Olecranon bursitis is usually traumatic, but the swelling can appear spontaneously. If pain is not a major feature, no treatment will be necessary, as resolution usually occurs in about one month. If pain, however, is a feature, but there no signs of infection, then fluid should be first aspirated and then 1ml. of Depomedrone injected into the site. If there are signs of infection, then aspiration only and treatment with oral antibiotics are indicated.

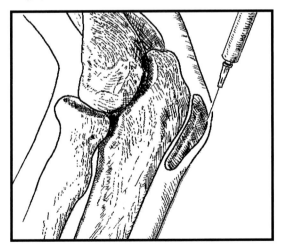

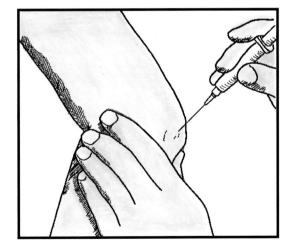

Figure 5.9 and 5.10 Injection for Olecranon Bursitis

WRIST

There are several painful conditions in the wrist for which treatment should be considered. Carpal tunnel syndrome is common in busy housewives. It usually resolves with splintage and rest. If it is persistent and severe, then surgical release may be necessary. In such cases it is worth trying first the effect of Depomedrone (1-2ml), injected just below the central point of the distal flexor crease at the wrist. It is important to take care not to inject into the median nerve.

Figure 5.11
Injection for Carpal Tunnel
Syndrome

De Quervain's tenosynovitis responds dramatically to Depomedrone injection. 0.5-1ml. is injected into the sheath of the extensor tendons at the radial styloid process.

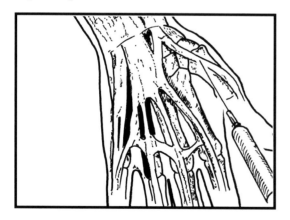 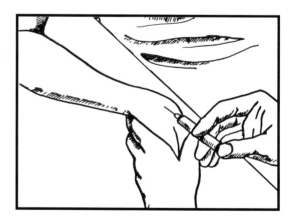

Figures 5.12 and 5.13 Injections for De Quervain's Tenosynovitis

Arthritis of carpo-metacarpal and metacarpo-phalangeal joints of the thumb and pain over the ulnar styloid also respond well to local injection of Depomedrone (1-2ml.).

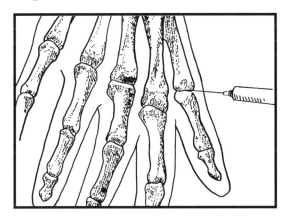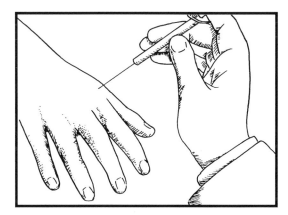

Figures 5.14 and 5.15 Injection for Arthritis

Ganglia are common on the dorsum of the wrist. They often resolve spontaneously, but if treatment is sought, then aspiration of the swelling with a large needle, with or without injection of Depomedrone (0.5ml.), may be curative.

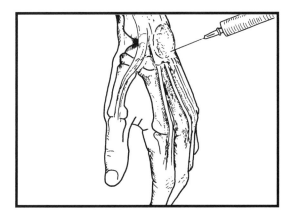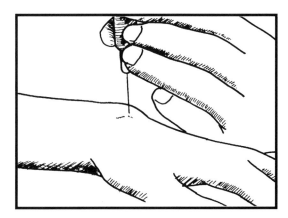

Figures 5.16 and 5.17 Injection for Ganglion

FINGERS

Trigger fingers may respond to Depomedrone (0.5ml.). The swelling of the affected tendon sheath tends to be over the metacarpo-phalangeal or inter-phalangeal joints. The injection of Depomedrone is placed into the swelling of the tendon sheath.

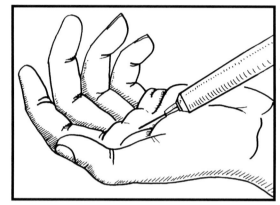

Figure 5.18
Injection for Trigger Finger

BACK

'Fibrositis' in the sacro-spinalis or gluteal region over the sacro-iliacs as denoted by tender nobules may be relieved by injections of Depomedrone (1-2ml.) and Xylocaine.

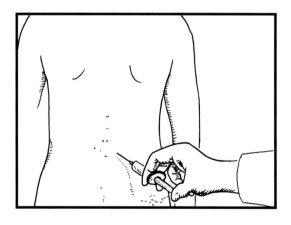

Figure 5.19
Injection for Fibrositis

KNEES

Several conditions of the knee respond well to injection with Depomedrone. Medial or lateral ligaments may become locally tender from minor trauma, and injection of 1-2ml. of Depomedrone can be dramatically effective in relieving pain and disability.

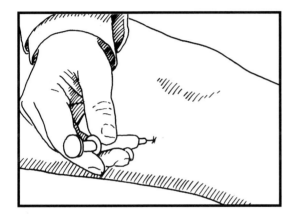

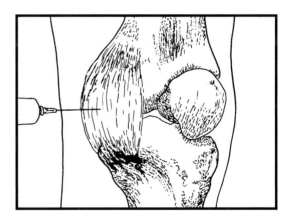

Figures 5.20 and 5.21
Injection for Minor Trauma
to Knee Ligaments

Osteo-arthritis of knee joints is very common in the elderly, especially overweight women, and also in men to a lesser extent. Treatment with analgesics, NSAIDs and physiotherapy is rarely successful. The injection of 2ml. of Depomedrone into the swollen knee joint may give considerable relief of pain. It is best to inject just above the patella laterally or medially. If it is effective, patients usually request further injections. These, however, should not be given more often than three monthly.

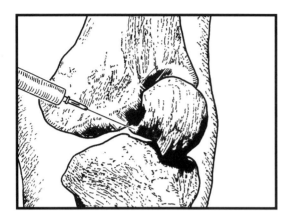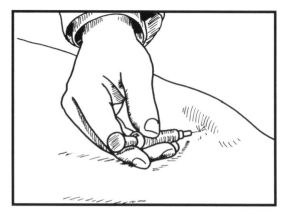

Figures 5.22 and 5.23 Injection for Osteo-Arthritis of the Knee Joint

Prepatellar bursitis, 'housemaid's knee', is now rare in women, but is an occupational condition of floor or road layers. The best treatment for this condition is to change jobs, but this is usually impossible. Aspiration of the effusion and injection with 1-2ml. of Depomedrone will be beneficial, accompanied by a period of rest.

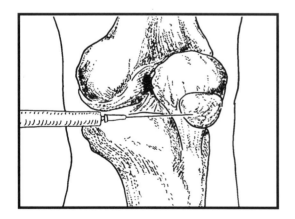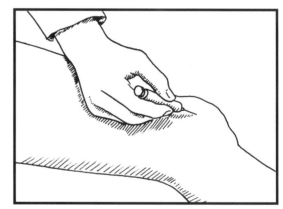

Figures 5.24 and 5.25 Injection for Prepatellar Bursitis

FEET

Painful heels with local tenderness over the calcaneum or at the insertion of the tendo achilles is an indication for injection of Depomedrone (0.5-1ml.) with Xylocaine 2% (0.5-1ml.). The procedure is painful but it can be very effective. It is important to take care not to inject into the tendo achilles itself.

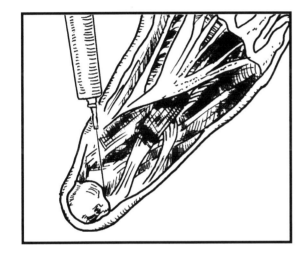

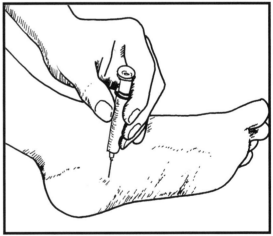

Figures 5.26 and 5.27
Injection for Painful Heels

GOUT AND RHEUMATOID ARTHRITIS

In cases of gout and rheumatoid arthritis, injections of Depomedrone into affected joints may relieve localised pain and swelling and can be of great benefit to the patient.

ANKLES

Post traumatic 'sprained ankles' may take many weeks to recover. If there is persistent localised tenderness over the lateral ligament, this can be an indication to try the effect of 1-2ml. of Depomedrone, which may give relief.

Ganglia in the ankle region should be managed in exactly the same manner as ganglia affecting the wrist.

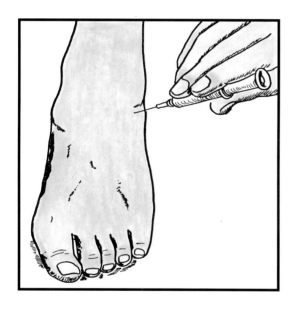

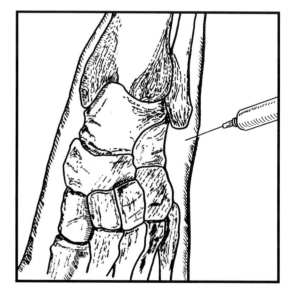

Figure 5.28 and 5.29
Injection for Sprained Ankle

Therapeutic Objectives

- injection of local steroids to control inflammatory reactions

- aspiration of fluids or blood from joint, bursa or ganglion to relieve tension

Diagnostic

- aspiration of fluid from joint for micro-organisms or crystals

Principles for Success of Injection of Steroids

- diagnostic accuracy

- sterility essential

- Depomedrone (methylprednisolone) is effective

- place injection in appropriate anatomical site

Chapter Six

Ear, Nose and Throat (ENT)

Much of modern ENT work requires special equipment and therefore the scope for procedures in general practice is limited. Those that are described, however, are practical and possible, providing that the following principles are observed. The equipment should be simple and flexible in usage. A good history is important, for instance in revealing possible contraindications, such as syringing an ear with a perforated drum. It is also important for the general practitioner to decide whether the procedure is within his or her capabilities.

The basic equipment needed is as follows:

- Otoscope with detachable lens and small swinging side-lens with a
- Side-channel for a Siegel's bulb.
- Aural speculae, which should include several of medium and large sizes. Small pinhole speculae are useless.
- Jobson Horne probes (2 or 3).
- Tilly's nasal dressing forceps.
- Lack's tongue depressors (various sizes).
- Thudicum's nasal speculae.
- Ribbon gauze (0.5" or 1").
- Tubes of B.I.P.P. (bismuth, iodoform and paraffin paste).
- Liquid paraffin.
- Silver nitrate sticks.
- Lignocaine spray and solution.

- Eustachian catheter (large bore).
- Higginson-type bulb syringe.
- Ear syringe - plastic or metal.
- Head mirror and a good light source.
- Henckel's fenestrated forceps.

EARS

There are certain conditions of the ear which can be safely treated by procedures in general practice. Wax is a natural secretion in the external meatus. Some people produce excess wax; in some the meatus is narrow and curved and wax, therefore, accumulates. This may cause hearing loss and when dry can predispose to external otitis. The aim of the treatment is to remove the wax safely and in comfort.

If the wax is hard, then it should be softened with an instillation of sodium bicarbonate ear drops (BNF) or almond or olive oil. If the wax is persistent, however, it can be removed by syringing (washing out) with warm tap water

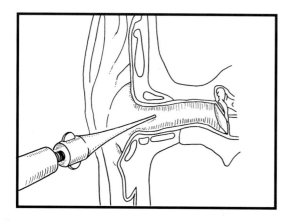

Figure 6.1
Syringing with Warm Tap Water

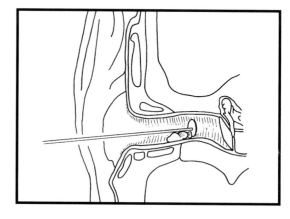

Figure 6.2
Removing Impacted Dry Wax with the
Ring of a Probe

using an ear syringe or Higginson-type syringe with attached Eustachian catheter. It is important not to syringe the ear if there is infection or perforation of the ear drum, or if there has been previous middle-ear surgery. Impacted dry wax may be gently lifted off the wall of the meatus by the ring of a probe, using the small otoscope lens, and then syringed out.

Foreign bodies in the external meatus may be removed by careful syringing. Foreign bodies may be of various materials, rough and smooth, soft and hard, and insects. Live insects should be first killed by the instillation of almond or olive oil. It is important to straighten the meatus by pulling the pinna up, back and in an outward direction. Ear syringing, in young children who are distressed, should be avoided. Attempts to syringe the ear of a fighting child spell humiliation and possible disaster. Unless the foreign body, such as polystyrene or cotton wool, is easily accessible, it is advisable not to attempt to remove it. It is important not to try and dig with forceps or probes. If the foreign body is inaccessible, the patient should be referred to an ENT unit.

When cleansing infected ears, there are various considerations to be taken into account. If there is pus or debris, this should be removed manually through an otoscope, using small pledgelets of cotton wool on a Jobson Horne

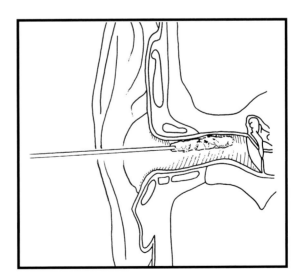

Figure 6.3
Removing Debris using
Jobson Horne Probe

probe. An intact drum signifies otitis externa; a perforation, otitis media. A perforated ear drum should not be syringed.

In severe otitis externa or in the case of a furuncle with oedema of the meatus, it is necessary to reduce the oedema. If this cannot be done by inserting astringent or steroid drugs, the oedema can be reduced by gently inserting a small wick of ribbon gauze soaked in aluminium acetate solution. One drop of the solution should be added to the exposed end of the wick every hour. The wick should be removed after twenty-four hours.

NOSE

There are various conditions in the nose which can be treated by the general practitioner. A good view of the inner nose can be obtained using an otoscope with the largest speculae and swing lens.

Foreign bodies are usually inserted by children. They tend to be soft materials such as paper, foam rubber or polystyrene. Local anaesthesia can be achieved by a lignocaine spray or a pledgelet of cotton wool soaked in it and inserted gently up the nose via the speculum. The foreign body can then be removed with Henckel's or Tilly's forceps. Repeated attempts are not recommended and if the procedure is unsuccessful referral to ENT is advisable.

Nose bleeds (epistaxis) in the young are from the anterior surface of the septum. Small bleeding vessels can be seen through the speculum and be cauterised with silver nitrate after local lignocaine anaesthesia. In the elderly, bleeding is often from the ethnoid region which is more posterior and packing may be necessary to control it. Ribbon gauze, soaked in lignocaine and adrenaline 1:1000, should be inserted for some four inches. After a few minutes, it should be replaced by a B.I.P.P. pack on both sides of the nose. If this does not control bleeding, referral to a hospital ENT unit is recommended.

Simple papillomata occur at the muco-cutaneous junction of the nasal vestibule. Small ones can be removed through repeated cauterisation with silver nitrate through a nasal speculum or an otoscope. Larger papillomata require diathermy or excision under general anaesthesia at hospital.

The removal of nasal polpi, antral washouts and intra-nasal biopsies should be undertaken at an ENT unit and not in general practice.

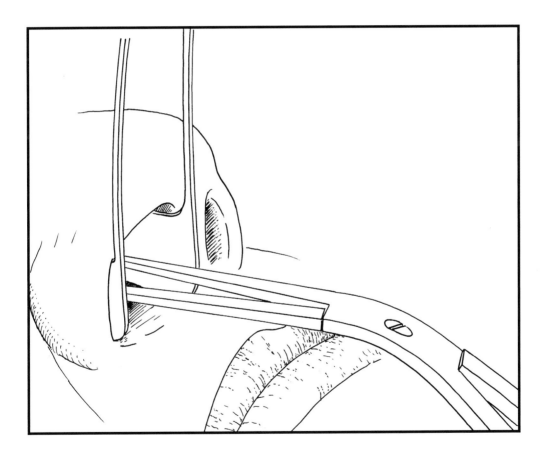

Figure 6.4 Removal of Foreign Body with Forceps

THROAT

Quinsy is a peritonsillar abscess with much local oedema and severe discomfort and toxicity. It is now rare and, when it does occur, it is most often in young adults. There should firstly be intensive treatment with antibiotics, probably intramuscular penicillin, to control and localise infection. Residual swelling denotes abscess formation that may require incision. This is usually best carried out in hospital under local anaesthesia with lignocaine 2% infiltration. In emergency situations, however, the abscess may need to be incised. The procedure, in this case, is to penetrate the mucosa with a Bard-Parker blade (size 15) and then the cavity should be opened with Tilly's nasal dressing forceps.

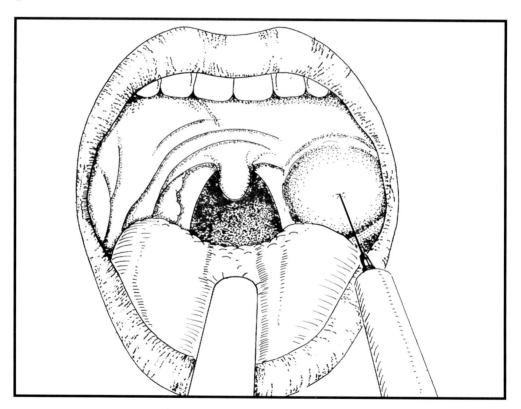

Figure 6.5 Local Anaesthetic Prior to Incision

Chapter Seven

Gynaecological Procedures

Gynaecology is very much part of general practice. Gynaecological examination and diagnosis are part of every day practice. All women with gynaecological symptoms should have an abdominal and pelvic examination carried out, including inspection of the vagina and cervix. The most useful speculum is the duck-billed, which may be sterilised or may be used as a disposable. The best form of lighting is from a good quality freestanding anglepoise lamp.

CERVICAL SMEAR AND IUD INSERTION AND REMOVAL

Cervical smear is a standard procedure. IUD insertion and removal should follow the instructions provided by the manufacturers.

CERVICAL EROSIONS

Not all erosions need treatment. Indications for treatment are persistent vaginal discharge and soreness and bleeding. All patients with cervical

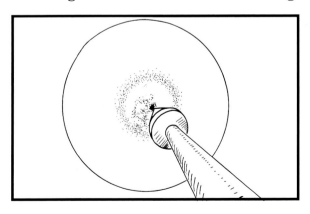

Figure 7.1
Treating Cervical Erosion by
Cryotherapy

erosions should have a cervical smear carried out and this should be repeated regularly. The best treatment in general practice is by cryocautery, if available, or by referral to a gynaecologist for electric diathermy.

CERVICAL POLYPS

Patients with large polyps should be referred for treatment at hospital. Small cervical polyps can be removed by twisting with sponge holding forceps and cauterising the base with silver nitrate. All cervical polyps which have been removed should be sent for histological examination.

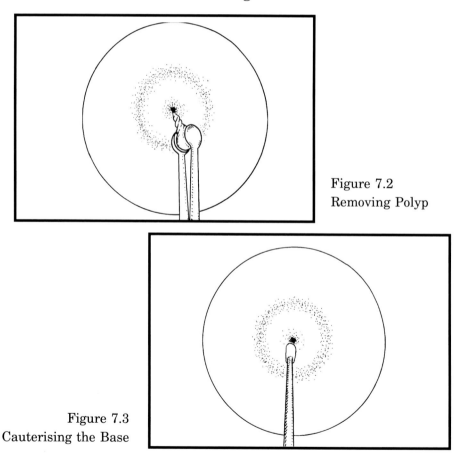

Figure 7.2
Removing Polyp

Figure 7.3
Cauterising the Base

GENITAL WARTS

If there is only a small number, then local applications of podophyllin solution are usually effective. If there are many warts, then the patient should be referred to hospital for diathermy under general anaesthesia. A cryoprobe can be used if one is available.

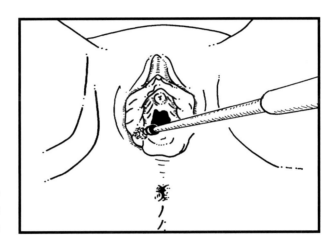

Figure 7.4
Treating Genital Wart
with Cryoprobe

HORMONE IMPLANTS

For hormone replacement therapy (HRT), a hormone implant can provide up to one year's treatment. An implant of oestradiol (100mg.) and testosterone (100mg.) is used. The sites for implantation are the upper outer quadrant of the buttock or the abdominal wall above the inguinal ligament. Firstly it is necessary to infiltrate the site to be used with local anaesthetic. Then a small incision should be made, to allow the trocar and cannula to be inserted. The trocar should then be removed and the requisite number of tablets inserted through the cannula into the subcutaneous space. The cannula should then be removed and a plaster applied.

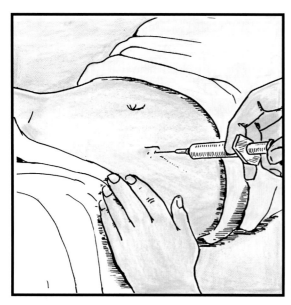

Figure 7.5
Injecting Local Anaesthetic

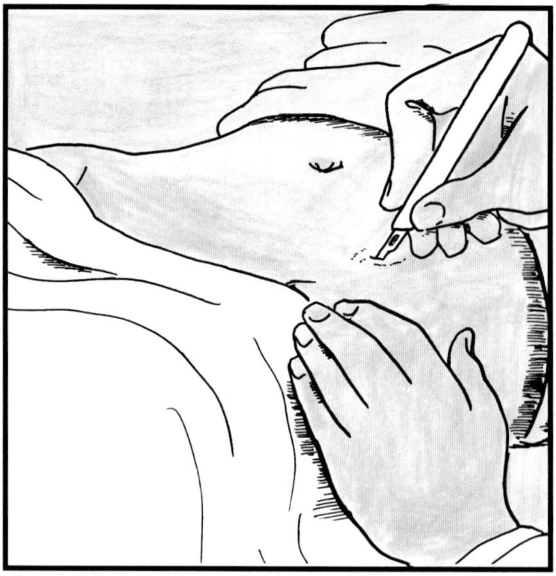

Figure 7.6
Incision for Trocar and Cannula

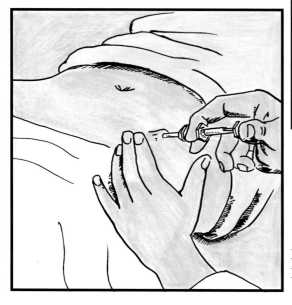

Figure 7.7
Inserting Trocar and Cannula

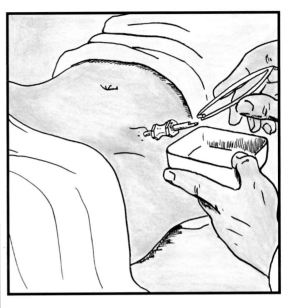

Figure 7.8
Inserting Tablet through Cannula

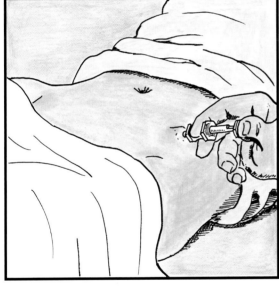

Figure 7.9
Replacing Trocar

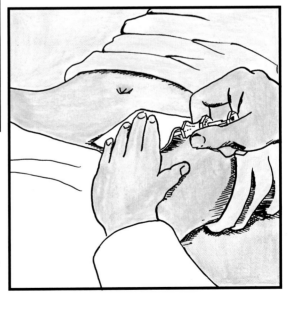

Figure 7.10
Removing Trocar and Cannula whilst
Applying Local Pressure

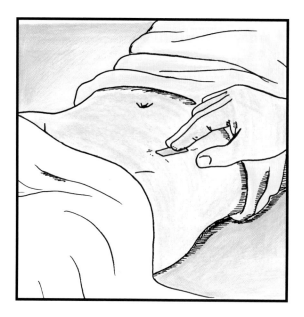

Figure 7.11 No Suture. Only Plaster Required

Colour Atlas of Minor Surgery in General Practice

Chapter Eight

Do's and Don'ts

AIDE MEMOIRE

Embarking, or re-embarking, on minor surgery in general practice is fraught with potential hazards that should be appreciated and can be avoided. We present here lists of some do's and don'ts.

DO'S

- Be prepared and trained and, if necessary, do not be ashamed to undertake a period of retraining.

- Ensure you have a good relationship with your local surgeons and be prepared to collaborate as often as is necessary with them.

- Confirm medico-legal safeguards with your defence organisation and follow Local Medical Committee advice on minor surgery in general practice.

- Limit your surgery to what is feasible and safe.

- Maintain an 'operations book' and keep good records of procedures and anaesthesia.

- Always work with an assistant.

- Provide adequate resources, equipment and facilities.

- Ensure effective sterilisation procedures, either on your practice premises or by obtaining sterile sets from the local hospital CSSD.

- Have facilities and equipment for emergency resuscitation and staff trained in its use.

- Send material removed for histological examination and report.

- Send swabs or samples of infected material or pus for bacteriological examination.

- Although X-rays of apparent minor injuries may not be indicated clinically, they may be required in possible medico-legal situations.

- Check on tetanus immunisation.

- Always arrange for a follow-up attendance.

- Carry out regular self-check audits on results, including complications, such as wound infection.

- Acknowledge mistakes when they occur.

DON'TS

- Don't undertake procedures which you are unable to carry out safely and effectively.

- Don't undertake procedures that may carry possible risks such as:
    Circumcision (in adults).
    Carpal tunnel release.
    Dissection of deep ganglia.
    Excision of hydrocoele.
    Ligation of saphenous veins in the groin.
    Searching for impalpable foreign bodies.
    Removal of embedded corneal foreign bodies.
    Syringing perforated ear drums.

- Don't operate alone.

- Don't work with inadequate resources or equipment.

- Don't use general anaesthesia unless carried out by a recognised anaesthetist.

- Don't treat piles without excluding possible cancer of the rectum or colon.

- Don't inject steroids 'blindly'.

- Don't be motivated by financial inducements.

Appendix

Further Reading

"Illustrated Handbook of Minor Surgery and Operative Technique"
Saleh and Sodera   Heinemann Medical Books

"Complications of Minor Surgery"   Stoddart & Smith   Bailliere Tindall

"Operating Theatre Technique"   Brigden R. J.   Churchill Livingstone

"Illustrated Handbook of Local Anaesthesia"   Eriksson E.   Lloyd Luke

"A Guide to Practical Procedures in Medicine and Surgery"   Dudley,
Eckersley and Paterson-Brown   Heinemann Medical Books

"General Surgery at the District Hospital"   Cook, Sankaran and Wasunna
World Health Organisation

"Minor Surgery, a Text and Atlas"   Brown   Chapman and Hall Medical

Appendix

Surgical Equipment - Retailers

Porter Nash Medical,
116, Wigmore Street,
London W1H 9FD

F. P Sales
28, Kelbourne Road
Cowley
Oxford OX4 3SZ

Philip Harris Medical
25, Gentlemans' Walk
Norwich NE2 1NA

Doctor Buying Service
13-21 High Street
Guildford GU1 3DX

GP Equipment
30, Lancaster Gate
London W2 3LP

Pulse Doctors Shop
Morgan Grampian House
Calderwood Street
London SE18 6QH

Bridge Medical Direct
118, Chatham Street
Reading RG1 7HT

Rocket of London
Imperial Way
Watford
Herts WD2 4XX

Seward Medical Ltd
131, Great Suffolk Street
London SE1 1PP

Key-Med Ltd
Key-Med House
Stock Road
Southend on Sea SS2 5QH

CryoService Ltd
Blackpole Trading Estate
Blackpole Road
Worcester WR3 8SG

Fern Developments Ltd.
7, Springburn Place
College Milton North
East Kilbride
Glasgow G74 5NU

INDEX